O A R L

OXFORD AMERICAN RHEUMATOLOGY LIBRARY

Fibromyalgia

O A R L

OXFORD AMERICAN RHEUMATOLOGY LIBRARY

Fibromyalgia

The Essential Clinician's Guide

Daniel J. Clauw, MD

Professor of Anesthesiology and Medicine
Associate Dean, Clinical and Translational Research
Director, Chronic Pain and Fatigue Research Center
University of Michigan Medical School
Ann Arbor, Michigan

Daniel J. Wallace, MD, FACP, FACR

Clinical Professor of Medicine
Division of Rheumatology
Cedars-Sinai Medical Center
David Geffen School of Medicine at UCLA
Los Angeles, California

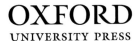

OXFORD

UNIVERSITY PRESS

OXFORD

UNIVERSITY PRESS

Oxford University Press, Inc., publishes works that further
Oxford University's objective of excellence
in research, scholarship, and education.

Oxford New York

Auckland Cape Town Dar es Salaam Hong Kong Karachi
Kuala Lumpur Madrid Melbourne Mexico City Nairobi
New Delhi Shanghai Taipei Toronto

With offices in
Argentina Austria Brazil Chile Czech Republic France Greece
Guatemala Hungary Italy Japan Poland Portugal Singapore
South Korea Switzerland Thailand Turkey Ukraine Vietnam

Published by Oxford University Press, Inc.
198 Madison Avenue, New York, New York 10016
www.oup.com

Oxford is a registered trademark of Oxford University Press

Library of Congress Cataloging-in-Publication Data
Wallace, Daniel J. (Daniel Jeffrey), 1949-
Fibromyalgia : the essential clinician's guide / Daniel J. Wallace, Daniel J. Clauw.
p. ; cm. – (Oxford American rheumatology library)
Includes bibliographical references.
ISBN 978-0-19-538441-3
1. Fibromyalgia.   I. Clauw, Daniel J.   II. Title.   III. Series.
[DNLM: 1. Fibromyalgia. WE 544 W188f 2008]
RC927.3.W345 2008
616.7'4–dc22   2008035016

9 8 7 6 5 4 3 2 1
Printed in USA
on acid-free paper

Acknowledgment

The authors acknowledge the assistance of Luba Goldin and Yvonne Honigsberg at Oxford University Press, our families, and support staffs at Cedars-Sinai Medical Center and the University of Michigan.

>

Contents

Chapter 1

History of fibromyalgia

Concepts of what is now regarded as fibromyalgia date to the Babylonian epic of Gilgamesh, the Bible ("and the days of affliction have taken hold upon me. My bones are pierced in the night season and my sinews take no rest." Job 30:16–17), and Shakespeare ("Therefore the moon, the governess of floods, pale in her anger, washes the air, that rheumatic diseases do abound." *A Midsummer Night's Dream*, Act 2, Scene 34, I, 105). The term *rheumatism* was first used by Guillaume de Bailou around 1592, and it was included in a 1763 glossary of rheumatic diseases by F. B. de Sauvages de la Croix.

Fibromyalgia represents a convergence of concepts, as shown in Table 1.1.[1] In other words, a similar clinical presentation ultimately evolved, and by the late 20th century it was apparent that these musculoskeletal manifestations of central pain or sensory augmentation represented a similar process.

Evolution of trigger and tender points

The British physician R. P. Player first described what are now regarded as tender points in 1821. They were described in more detail by F. Villeix in an 1841 treatise ("points douloureaux"). Additional insights derived in the 19th century include its predilection for females, the presence of nodules, associated muscular spasm, pain, stiffness, and somatic complaints. Sir William R. Gowers (1845–1915) coined the term *fibrositis* in a paper on lumbago (low back pain) in 1904. Sir Thomas Lewis and Jonas Kellgren mapped out tender and trigger pains as well as referred pain patterns in the 1930s. Arthur Steindler demonstrated amelioration of local symptoms with procaine injections in 1937. Janet Travell (1901–1997) was the

Table 1.1 Fibromyalgia: A convergence of concepts
• Trigger and tender points
• Neurasthenia
• Postinfectious fatigue syndromes
• Chronic widespread pain in wartime
• Myalgic encephalomyelitis
• Myasthenic syndrome
• Post-traumatic myofascial pain
• "Continuous" trauma

White House physician to John F. Kennedy and Lyndon B. Johnson. She elaborated on these findings and is thought to be largely responsible for founding the discipline now known as physical medicine. In part because of a differing philosophy regarding the underlying pathophysiology, there has been a gradual divergence between what the terms *tender point* (an area of the body that displays increased tenderness upon palpation—the number of which is a measure, albeit poor, of an individual's overall pain sensitivity) and *trigger points* (a regional phenomenon accompanied by the presence of "taut bands" and referred pain).

Neurasthenia

The state of "nervous exhaustion," or chronic fatigue, was first studied by Austin Flint in the early 1800s and detailed by George Beard (1839–1883), who coined the term *neurasthenia,* and Silas Weir Mitchell (1829–1914), who "packaged" the condition in the United States and treated it with a combination of Faradic currents and misogynistic approaches (e.g., removal of the clitoris, encouraging masturbation via horseback riding). Neurasthenia was the longest section in the 1899 edition of Sir William Osler's textbook of medicine. The term largely disappeared after World War I.

Postinfectious fatigue syndromes

The association between established infections and psychological or fatigue states was attributed to malaria or "wasting fevers" in the 1860s and typhoid fever by Osler, among others. In the 1930s and 1940s reports of postinfectious fatigue syndromes were published relating to polio and brucellosis. In the 1970s, chronic fatigue was attributed to yeast and the Epstein-Barr virus, but rigorous study methods suggested that this either did not occur or was not limited to these microbes. Ultimately, terminology used by infectious disease and internal medicine specialists was refined by the Centers for Disease Control in their 1988 classification for defining cases of "chronic fatigue syndrome."

Chronic widespread pain in wartime

Complaints of chronic fatigue or musculoskeletal pain in wartime date back to the 1700s but were first documented in British pensioners after the Crimean War (1853–1856). "Effort syndrome" or "irritable heart" was noted by Jacob da Costa, a Union surgeon during the U.S. Civil War (1861–1865), where fatigue, difficulty sleeping, palpitations, digestive disturbances, and headache required removal from the battlefield. Six hundred thousand cases of "da Costa's syndrome" were noted by the British military during the World War I. In 1942, 69% of all referrals to British military hospitals were for "fibrositis," which also included difficulty in carrying weaponry. Post-traumatic stress disorder (PTSD) was associated with musculoskeletal complaints in soldiers in the U.S. military during the Vietnam War (1961–1975) and the Iraq conflicts. Postwar somatic syndromes are not confined to wars that are accompanied by intensely stressful events; in the first Gulf War there was very little PTSD but still a very high rate of postdeployment chronic widespread pain, fatigue, memory difficulties, and so forth.

Myalgic encephalomyelitis

Also known as epidemic neuromyasthenia and myalgic encephalomyelitis, this English terminology was applied to "outbreaks" of fibromyalgia after polio or other infectious epidemics between 1934 and 1987. Sometimes the onset of these events was associated with mass hysteria; chronicity of symptoms was a common feature.

Myasthenic syndrome

Before rheumatology was a recognized subspecialty and access to a rheumatology consultant was generally available, many individuals with fibromyalgia were diagnosed by neurologists between 1930 and 1965 as having "myasthenic syndrome," or myasthenia gravis–like symptoms with a negative Tensilon test. Interestingly, many of these patients were pre-scribed pyridostigmine with favorable responses, which led the University of Oregon to recently report that this agent had effects similar to growth hormone.

Post-traumatic myofascial pain

In 1866, a London surgeon, John E. Erichsen (1818–1896), described "railway spine" as a form of post-traumatic back pain that was more severe and of longer duration than expected from the attributable injury (Fig. 1.1). A Los Angeles orthopedist, H. D. Crowe, described eight cases of post–automobile accident neck pain in 1928 and coined the term *whiplash*. Widespread chronic musculoskeletal pain was reported in some of those cases. Legal considerations have made it difficult to separate science from fact in this area, but these patients have been shown to have widespread tenderness and hyperalgesia, just as is seen in fibromyalgia.

"Continuous trauma" and fibromyalgia

Myofascial pain among Welsh coal miners stemming from repeated heavy lifting was officially recognized by the British government as a compens-able injury in the 1920s as "worker's compensation" insurance plans were becoming widespread. This phenomenon was subject to considerable abuse, as exemplified by the "epidemic" of "repetitive strain syndrome" among Australian workers in the 1980s that largely disappeared after

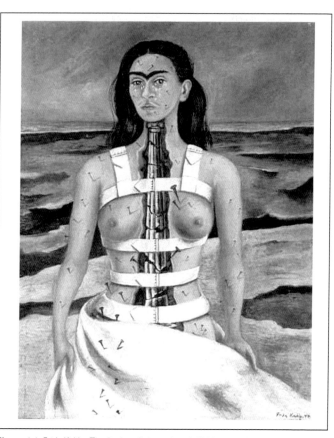

Figure 1.1 Frida Kahlo: The Broken Column (1916). Kahlo painted numerous self-portraits expressing the chronic pain she suffered subsequent to a bus accident. Reproduced with permission from Museo Dolores Olmedo Patiño, Mexico City, Mexico.

regulatory terminology was changed. Pre-employment psychological profiles and musculoskeletal complaints may play a role in predicting which employees with certain job descriptions will develop symptoms and seek compensation for their plight. The role of continuous trauma is nevertheless a real one, and many of these individuals develop fibromyalgia.

Summary: The convergence of concepts

Work in the 1970s by Hugh Smythe and colleagues at the University of Toronto connected the musculoskeletal complaints with poor sleep and tender points.[2] Muhammad Yunus and colleagues at the University of Illinois in the 1980s renamed fibrositis as *fibromyalgia* and associated the above with somatic complaints and other functional syndromes. This led the American Medical Association to opine in 1987 that fibromyalgia syndrome represented a distinct entity.[3] An ad hoc committee of the American College of Rheumatology formulated and validated criteria for fibromyalgia syndrome in 1990, and the concept was endorsed by the Copenhagen declaration of the World Health Organization in 1992.

References

1. Wallace DJ. The history of fibromyalgia. In Wallace DJ, Clauw DJ, eds. *Fibromyalgia and Other Central Pain Syndromes*. Philadelphia: Lippincott Williams & Wilkins; 2005:1–8.

2. Smythe H. Fibrositis syndrome: a historical perspective. *J Rheumatol*. 1989;16(Supp 19):2–6.

3. Bennett RM. Fibromyalgia. *JAMA*. 1987;257:2802–2803.

Chapter 2

Definitions and classification

Fibromyalgia is not a discrete disease but rather a syndrome or construct. The term was first suggested by Kahler Hench in 1976 and adopted by Yunus in his 1980s studies, which suggested that systemic and somatic complaints were statistically associated with myofascial tenderness. A 1987 editorial in the *Journal of the American Medical Association* suggested that a validated definition for fibromyalgia would be useful, and this led to the formation of an ad hoc committee. Its findings were published in 1990. All the terms defined in this chapter are elaborated on in other chapters of this monograph.

The 1990 classification criteria for fibromyalgia

A multicenter criteria committee led by Frederick Wolfe studied 558 consecutive patients, 293 with fibromyalgia and 265 controls. A combination of widespread pain (pain in all four quadrants of the body and the axial skeleton) with tenderness in at least 11 of 18 tender point sites (when 4 kg of pressure is applied) of at least 3 months' duration, with other etiologies being excluded, yielded a sensitivity of 88.4% and a specificity of 81.1%.[1] This is shown in Table 2.1 and Figure 2.1. The American College of Rheumatology (ACR) endorsed the committee's recommendations. These classification criteria, intended for use in research studies but not meant to be used to diagnose individual patients, have allowed the science of fibromyalgia to rapidly evolve since 1990.

Failings and misuse of the criteria

There are many problems with the ACR criteria, especially when they are misused and applied to individual patients in clinical practice. These include the following:

- They assume that the pain thresholds for women and men are similar, and thus use the same threshold of 11 tender points as being indicative of fibromyalgia in both women and men. In fact, women are much more sensitive to pain, using any type of experimental pain testing, than men. Thus we should either apply greater pressure or accept lower numbers of tender points to consider a male tender, and this would lead to more males being appropriately diagnosed with fibromyalgia.

- We now know that fibromyalgia patients are tender throughout the entire body, not just in these 18 locations. In fact, we now know that tender points are merely areas of the body where one is more tender. The difference between the pain threshold of a fibromyalgia patient and that of a control is just as great in areas such as the thumbnail and forehead as in regions considered to be tender points, so one can push anywhere in the body to assess pain threshold.

- Tender points are not a good measure of pressure pain threshold, since the number of tender points an individual displays is in part related to his or her pain threshold and in part related to distress levels. More sophisticated measures of experimental pain or sensory testing are far superior to counting tender points in assessing an individual's overall pain or sensory threshold.

Also, although the criteria have been validated by other surveys, the ACR classification focuses only on pain. It ignores important fibromyalgia symptoms such as fatigue, cognitive disturbance, alterations in sleep architecture, and psychological distress, as well as commonly associated syndromes such as irritable bowel syndrome. Further, the legal community has taken a narrow view of the criteria in applying them to litigation, which ignores the considerations enumerated in the beginning of this paragraph.

Chronic widespread pain

A highly respected epidemiologic unit in Manchester, United Kingdom, addressed some of the failings of the ACR criteria and was concerned that cases of clinically meaningful widespread pain could be excluded. Their definition of "chronic widespread pain" differs from the ACR "four quadrant" one in that it requires more diffuse limb pain, present in two or more sections of contralateral limbs, and axial pain present for 3 months. These individuals have more severe disability and higher levels of associated symptoms.[2] Chronic widespread pain is also often present without tender points.

Table 2.1 ACR 1990 criteria for the classification of fibromyalgia

1. History of widespread pain; must include all four quadrants of the body and axial skeletal pain.

2. Pain in 11 of 18 tender point sites with at least 4 kg of pressure on digital palpation. These sites are in occipital, low cervical, trapezius, supraspinatus, second rib, lateral epicondyle, gluteal, greater trochanter, and anserine knee bursal regions as shown in Figure 2.1.

3. Both the above criteria must be present for at least 3 months provided a second clinical disorder does not exclude the diagnosis. For a tender point to be considered positive, the subject must state that the palpation was painful. "Tender" is not to be considered "painful."

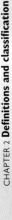

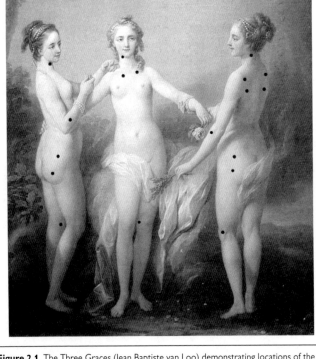

Figure 2.1 The Three Graces (Jean Baptiste van Loo) demonstrating locations of the tender points mentioned in Table 2.1. Reproduced with permission from Chateau de Chenonceau, Chenonceaux, France.

Regional myofascial pain (myofascial pain syndrome)

There is considerable controversy regarding the existence of myofascial pain as a discrete entity. On one end of the continuum are many who feel that myofascial pain may be a pathophysiology distinct from fibromyalgia and may represent a local muscle process. At the other end of the continuum are others (including the authors) who feel that in many or even most cases, myofascial pain is merely a regional form of fibromyalgia. Regional myofascial pain patients tend to include more males, and cases tend to be related to work or repetitive tasks.

We will not try to resolve this controversy but would suggest that patients with myofascial pain may respond well to the therapies suggested for fibromyalgia; conversely, if a patient has primarily regional pain and does not display more "systemic" features, such as diffuse tenderness, fatigue, memory problems, and pain elsewhere in the body, these individuals may benefit from local therapies that have been shown to be of value in myofascial pain. Also, since we know that a significant minority of patients with regional pain can develop widespread pain (likely via processes such as central sensitization), it is important to treat regional pain aggressively to attempt to prevent this from occurring.

Central sensitivity syndrome

Central sensitivity syndromes (CSS), a term coined by Yunus, is a category used to describe all syndromes characterized by failure to adequately dampen sensory afferent signals, with a resultant amplification of pain.[3] Although this term has not gained wide acceptance, the underlying construct is the same as that proposed by advocates of terms such as functional somatic syndromes, somatization, chronic multisymptom illnesses, medically unexplained syndromes, and so forth.

The reason we prefer to use the term CSS in this book is that at present it seems to give the most accurate information regarding the underlying pathophysiology of these illnesses. Nearly all of the conditions within this spectrum have been shown to be characterized by hypersensitivity to pain (e.g., performing experimental pain testing and identifying widespread hyperalgesia [increased pain to normally nonpainful stimuli] and allodynia [pain in response to normally nonpainful stimuli]). In most of these conditions there are also data suggesting a more global problem with hypersensitivity to any type of sensory stimuli, and we are beginning to understand the neurobiology of this phenomenon (and the neurobiology is independent of psychological factors). Most patients with fibromyalgia have a personal history of at least one and usually more of these associated syndromes, and these conditions are very familial and genetic, so it is common to see individuals whose family members have a history of regional and widespread pain (see Chapter 4 for pathogenesis). These entities can be regional or systemic and are listed in Table 2.2.

Outdated terminology

The following terms have been used historically to describe some of the above conditions but no longer have any meaningful validity: myofasciitis, fibrositis, neurasthenia, myalgic encephalomyelitis, and myositis with normal muscle enzyme levels.

Summary

Fibromyalgia is a form of chronic widespread pain with diffuse tenderness. Individuals who eventually develop fibromyalgia often have a history of other regional syndromes that fall under the umbrella of "central sensitivity

Table 2.2 Examples of some Central *Sensitivity* syndromes

- Fibromyalgia
- Myofascial pain syndrome
  - Temporomandibular disorder
  - Whiplash
  - Repetitive strain disorder
  - Chronic idiopathic low back pain
- Chronic fatigue syndrome; postinfectious fatigue syndromes
- Gastrointestinal syndromes
  - Non-ulcer dyspepsia
  - Esophageal dysmotility
  - Irritable bowel syndrome
  - Biliary dyskinesia; post-cholecystectomy syndrome
- Cardiac region syndromes
  - Syndrome X
  - Non-cardiac chest pain
  - Costochondritis
  - Mitral valve prolapse
- Headache: tension-type, migraine
- Gynecologic syndromes
  - Primary dysmenorrhea
  - Chronic pelvic pain
  - Dyspareunia, vulvodynia, vulvovestibulitis
  - Endometriosis
- Urologic syndromes
  - Irritable bladder/painful bladder
  - Interstitial cystitis
  - Chronic prostatitis
- Psychiatric conditions
  - Depression/anxiety
  - Post-traumatic stress disorder
  - Bipolar illness
- Multiple chemical sensitivities (a form of anxiety)
- Periodic limb movement disorder
- Dysautonomias

syndromes." Recent evidence suggests that there is neurobiological evidence of pain and sensory amplification in these disorders. In addition, prominent psychological, social, and cognitive factors play a role in symptom expression in these illnesses. An understanding of the confluence of factors that can lead to symptom expression gives the underpinning for an effective management strategy for these patients.

References

1. Wolfe F, Smythe HA, Yunus MB, et al. The American College of Rheumatology criteria for the classification of fibromyalgia. Report of the multicenter criteria committee. *Arthritis Rheum*. 1990;33:160–172.

2. Macfarlane GJ, Croft PR, Schollum J, et al. Widespread pain: is an improved classification possible? *J Rheumatol.* 1996;23:1628–1632.

3. Yunus MB. Central sensitivity syndromes: a new paradigm and group nosology for fibromyalgia and overlapping conditions, and the related issue of disease versus illness. *Semin Arthritis Rheum.* 2008; Jan 11 [E-pub ahead of print].

Chapter 3

Epidemiology

Pain has many etiologies, which fall into nociceptive (i.e., inflammation or damage of peripheral tissues), neuropathic (damage to nerves), and idiopathic or central pain. A form of chronic widespread pain, fibromyalgia falls into the last grouping. Surveys have suggested that 10% of citizens of developed countries have chronic widespread pain and 20% have chronic regional pain. In the United States, approximately 10% to 15% of the population has pain symptoms severe enough to seek medical attention.[1–4]

How many people have fibromyalgia?

Approximately one person in 50 in the United States fulfills the ACR criteria for fibromyalgia. Eighty percent to 90% are females, with a probable prevalence of 34/1000 females and 5/1000 males.[4] This difference in prevalence in females and males is largely due to the fact that very few males with chronic widespread pain also have 11 or greater tender points, but women are only 1.5 times as likely as men to have chronic widespread pain.

Prevalence estimates vary widely depending of the method of ascertainment used. This could be a postal survey, a health plan coding inventory, or a hospital discharge diagnosis or clinic population. For example, one epidemiologic survey concluded that 10% of Norwegians have fibromyalgia, while another in neighboring Denmark found a prevalence of 0.66%.

Fibromyalgia is estimated to be the second to fourth most common reason that an individual consults a rheumatologist. Some individuals never seek medical attention for their complaints but at a health fair or routine unsolicited screen turn out to fulfill the ACR criteria. They have what is known as *community fibromyalgia*, and at present there are probably at least as many undiagnosed as diagnosed cases of fibromyalgia. Hence, there are probably at a minimum 5 million, and possibly up to 15 million, Americans with fibromyalgia.

Who develops fibromyalgia?

Patients between the ages of 30 and 49 represent 60% of diagnosed cases; 35% are in their 20s or between the ages of 50 and 65 at the time of diagnosis.[3] In addition to a female predominance (because of a bias in the definition requiring a certain number of tender points, and since women also have more pain than men), certain work groups are preferentially affected.

In one survey, the prevalence of fibromyalgia was almost zero in professional workers, 0.5% in those employed in industry, 0.8% in service workers, 1.5% in agriculture, and 1.9% in those never employed. Risk factors for developing fibromyalgia include poor sleep, psychological distress, smoking, fatigue, anxiety, a family history of fibromyalgia, and the presence of any of the associated syndromes listed in Table 2.2.

Can animals develop fibromyalgia?

Numerous studies have documented tender points and lameness in dogs and other animals, but veterinary textbooks do not use the word *fibromyalgia*. There are, however, innumerable animal models of hyper-algesia/allodynia, the neurophysiological equivalent of fibromyalgia. Many of the triggers of fibromyalgia in humans (e.g., trauma, peripheral pain due to damage or inflammation) have been shown to lead to this hyperalgesic state in animals.

Primary vs. secondary fibromyalgia: Are there inciting factors?

Although there is no difference clinically, the term *primary fibromyalgia* has often historically been used to denote individuals who do not attribute the syndrome's onset to any particular event or inciting factor. Although the majority of fibromyalgia patients make no causative attribution, over 50 medical circumstances have been associated with bringing on the syndrome.

Single-event trauma

Physical trauma is undisputedly associated with post-event localized pain.[2] In some individuals, this regional pain fails to resolve and in fact becomes more widespread and chronic. The rate at which regional pain syndromes such as whiplash convert to chronic widespread pain differs markedly from country to country. Although it would be appealing to assume that these difference are due to differences in disability and litigation systems within different countries, this does not seem to be the case, as this occurs commonly in countries with "no fault" and/or national health insurance. Unfortunately, controversies regarding the social and political issues involved in litigation and compensation often distract clinicians, and they "throw the baby out with the bathwater," ignoring the overwhelming data that fibromyalgia is "real" because they do not believe patients are "worthy" of being eligible for these processes.

The authors wish to emphasize a few points:

• Ninety percent of post-traumatic myofascial pain resolves within 3 months if there is no serious injury (e.g., fracture, shock).

- A review of a prior medical record or history in patients who claim new onset of myofascial pain or fibromyalgia reveals evidence of a central sensitivity syndrome in the overwhelming majority, although it may not have been labeled as such. The court system can decide whether this is still a "compensable" injury in this setting.
- True "post-traumatic fibromyalgia" should be considered only when there is a close temporal relationship between regional pain that is due to trauma and the subsequent development of more widespread pain. Even then it is not clear that this term should be used clinically, because the prognosis may be worse in individuals who believe that their fibromyalgia was caused by someone or something else.
- Long-standing, chronic widespread pain with tender points (fibromyalgia) after a trivial injury may occur, but this is extremely rare.
- A preexisting fibromyalgia or myofascial pain syndrome can be aggravated by trauma and many other types of "stress."

Continuous trauma

Repetitive heavy lifting, pulling, bending, stooping, squatting, or strains (e.g., brought on by excessive keyboarding hand use), among other activities, may lead to regional myofascial pain. If not adequately addressed, a few of these individuals may develop fibromyalgia. Unfortunately, these complaints are confounded when made part of a worker's compensation complaint by a variety of factors, which are reviewed in Chapter 12.

Postinfectious fatigue syndromes

Some infections induce profound fatigue that becomes chronic, even after the infection has resolved. Some examples of infections that can trigger fibromyalgia include viral hepatitis, Epstein-Barr virus, Lyme disease, parvovirus, and human immunodeficiency virus. Some of these patients also experience joint aches, have tender points, and are diagnosed with fibromyalgia. This overlaps with chronic fatigue syndrome (see Chapter 7).

Inflammation- or medication-related fibromyalgia

A relatively high percentage (up to 20%) of patients with inflammatory conditions such as rheumatoid arthritis or systemic lupus erythematosus have or subsequently develop fibromyalgia. When this occurs, patients need to be treated for both the inflammatory disease and the fibromyalgia. Also, some anti-inflammatory regimens (e.g., corticosteroids, alpha-interferon) can produce hyperesthesia, aching, or cognitive changes associated with fibromyalgia.

Psychological stress and distress

Although there is no question that psychological stress may sometimes trigger or exacerbate fibromyalgia, not all "stress" seems to be equally capable of doing this, and not all people with "stress" develop chronic widespread pain or fibromyalgia. For example, population-based studies show that individuals with high levels of distress (but no pain) in the population are about twice as likely to develop chronic widespread pain as those without distress. However, even though there is a higher relative risk, the overwhelming majority of new cases of chronic widespread pain in the community *did not* have high levels of distress at baseline.

With respect to the type of stress that can best trigger or exacerbate these illnesses, it seems as though interpersonal stressors are the most likely. On the other hand, community stressors such as the terrorist attacks of 9/11 did not seem to lead to a higher rate of fibromyalgia in the population of New York City or worsen preexisting fibromyalgia in patients in Washington, D.C.

Finally, patients with a history of nearly any type of psychiatric disorder have an increased likelihood of developing fibromyalgia, and individuals with fibromyalgia are also more likely to develop many types of psychiatric disorders. This is consistent with data showing a weak shared familial predisposition for psychiatric disorders and fibromyalgia and related syndromes. This likely occurs because genetic abnormalities involving the breakdown or activity of neurotransmitters that are involved in both psychiatric disorders and pain (e.g., serotonin, norepinephrine, substance P) lead to a higher rate of both types of disorders, and because "stress" can trigger both types of disorders.

This theoretical link between stress, changes in stress axis activity, and subsequent susceptibility to somatic symptoms or syndromes is also supported by studies showing that patients with fibromyalgia and related conditions may be more likely than nonaffected individuals to have experienced physical or sexual abuse in childhood. Twin studies have recently supported a link between PTSD and trauma and chronic widespread pain. A recent study of Israeli war veterans with PTSD showed that those who exercised regularly were much less likely to develop chronic widespread pain or fibromyalgia.

Summary

At least 2% of the population of nearly any country or culture has fibromyalgia. Most individuals diagnosed at present are women who were diagnosed in their 30s or 40s, but ideally more males and younger individuals with the condition will be diagnosed as clinicians become more comfortable with making this diagnosis. While the inciting factor that brings on fibromyalgia is often not known, stressors such as trauma, psychological distress, infections, inflammation, or medication can antedate many cases.

References

1. Wallace DJ, Wallace JB. *Fibromyalgia: An Essential Guide to Patients and Their Families.* New York/London: Oxford University Press; 2003:8–13.

2. McLean S, Clauw DJ, Williams DA. The role of trauma in chronic neuromuscular pain. In Wallace DJ, Clauw DJ. *Fibromyalgia and Other Central Pain Syndromes.* Philadelphia: Lippincott Williams & Wilkins; 2005:267–279.

3. White KP, Speechley M, Harth M, et al. The London Fibromyalgia Epidemiology Study: Comparing the demographic and clinical characteristics in 100 random community cases of fibromyalgia versus controls. *J Rheumatol.* 1999;26:885–889.

4. Wolfe F, Ross K, Anderson J, et al. The prevalence and characteristics of fibromyalgia in the general population. *Arthritis Rheum.* 1995;38:19–28.

Chapter 4

Etiology and pathogenesis

Fibromyalgia is a central *sensitivity* syndrome characterized by increased responsiveness to sensory afferent stimuli, which results in pain amplification. To understand what goes awry in fibromyalgia, we will first provide a focused review of normal pain pathways.

Thermal, electrical, tactile, chemical, and other stimuli are processed by the sensory afferent system. This information is transmitted to the dorsal root ganglion of the spinal column by A-delta fibers (fast, myelinated), A-beta fibers (which carry tactile-mediated signals), C fibers (thin, unmyelinated, slow; carry dull sensations), and B fibers (autonomically mediated). These impulses are modulated in the spinal column by excitatory amino acids (e.g., NMDA, glutamate), substance P, nerve growth factor, and other chemicals, which ultimately are sent to the thalamus via the spinothalamic tract (except for autonomic impulses, which are transmitted via the spinoreticular system) and many other pathways. Noxious stimuli induce a specific cerebral cortical response that dampens pain by releasing a variety of neurotransmitters such as serotonin, norepinephrine, and endorphins.

In 1965, Melzack and Wall proposed the gate theory of pain, in which inhibitory pathways can block the propagation of excess sensory afferent signals by "closing the gate" under certain circumstances. Central sensitization syndromes occur when these defenses are overwhelmed. A variety of clinical abnormalities can ensue, from increased nociceptive input leading to more pain that would be expected from a painful stimulus (hyperpathia), normally nonpainful stimuli producing pain (allodynia), or autonomic B fibers carrying information from overloaded C and A fibers (dysautonomias). As will be discussed, several mechanisms are responsible for this.

Genetic factors

Research has indicated a strong familial component to the development of fibromyalgia. First-degree relatives of individuals with fibromyalgia have an eight-fold greater risk of developing fibromyalgia than those in the general population.[1] These studies also show that family members of individuals with fibromyalgia are much more tender than the family members of controls, regardless of whether they have pain or not. Family members of fibromyalgia patients are also much more likely to have irritable bowel syndrome, temporomandibular dysfunction, headaches, and a host of other regional pain syndromes. This familial and personal co-aggregation of conditions that includes fibromyalgia was originally collectively termed *affective spectrum disorder*, and more recently *central sensitivity syndromes* and *chronic multisymptom illnesses*. In population-based studies, the key symptoms that often co-aggregate besides pain are fatigue, memory difficulties, and mood disturbances. Twin studies suggest that approximately half of the risk of developing chronic widespread pain is due to genetic factors, and the other half is environmental.

Recent studies have begun to identify specific genetic polymorphisms that are associated with a higher risk of developing fibromyalgia. To date, the serotonin 5-HT2A receptor polymorphism T/T phenotype, serotonin transporter, dopamine 4 receptor, and COMT (catecholamine-O-methyl transferase) polymorphisms have all been seen in higher frequency in fibromyalgia.[2] All of the polymorphisms identified to date involve the metabolism or transport of monoamines, compounds that play a critical role in activity of the human stress response. It is likely that there are scores of genetic polymorphisms, involving other neuromodulators as well as monoamines, which in part determine an individual's set point for pain and sensory processing.

Pathogenesis

Role of stressors

Once fibromyalgia develops, the mechanisms responsible for ongoing symptom expression are likely complex and multifactorial. Because of the fact that disparate stressors can trigger the development of these conditions, the human stress response has been closely examined for a causative role. These systems are mediated primarily by the activity of the corticotropin-releasing hormone nervous system located in the hypothalamus and the locus ceruleus–norepinephrine/autonomic (sympathetic/LC-NE) nervous system in the brain stem. Recent research suggests that although this system in humans has been highly adaptive throughout history, the stress response may be inappropriately triggered by a wide assortment of everyday occurrences that do not pose a real threat to survival, thus initiating the cascade of physiologic responses more frequently than can be tolerated.[3]

Role of neuroendocrine abnormalities

Because of this link between exposure to stressors and the subsequent development of fibromyalgia, the human stress systems have been extensively studied in this condition. These studies have generally shown alterations of the hypothalamic-pituitary-adrenal (HPA) axis and the sympathetic nervous system in fibromyalgia and related conditions.[4,5] Although these studies often note either hypo- or hyperactivity of both the HPA axis and sympathetic nervous system in individuals with fibromyalgia and related conditions, the precise abnormality varies from study to study. Moreover, these studies find "abnormal" HPA axis or autonomic function in only a very small percentage of patients, and there is tremendous overlap between patients and controls in any of these studies.

It is likely that these neurobiological alterations are shared with other syndromes that are known to be associated with HPA and/or autonomic function, such as depression or PTSD. A model of susceptibility and development of these disorders that takes into account both genetics and personality as risk factors is illustrated in Figure 4.1. This recognizes the critical importance of stressors in resetting stress response systems, as well as other factors, including (1) the role of behavioral adaptations to these stressors, such as cessation of routine exercise, and (2) whether an individual is in an environment characterized by control or support.

Augmented pain and sensory processing as hallmarks of fibromyalgia and related syndromes

Once fibromyalgia is established, by far the most consistently detected objective abnormalities involve pain and sensory processing systems. Since fibromyalgia is defined in part by tenderness, considerable work has been performed exploring the potential reason for this phenomenon. The results of two decades of psychophysical pressure pain testing in fibromyalgia have been very instructive. One of the earliest findings in this regard was that the tenderness in fibromyalgia is not confined to tender points; instead it extends throughout the entire body. Theoretically, such diffuse tenderness could be primarily due to either psychological (e.g., hypervigilance, where individuals are too attentive to their surroundings) or neurobiological (e.g., the plethora of factors that can lead to temporary or permanent amplification of sensory input) factors.

Early studies typically used dolorimetry to assess pressure pain threshold and concluded that tenderness was in large part related to psychological factors, because these measures of pain threshold were correlated with levels of distress. To minimize the biases associated with "ascending" (i.e., the individual knows that the pressure will be predictably increased)

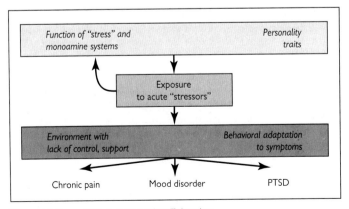

Figure 4.1 Susceptibility to "stress-related" disorders.

measures of pressure pain threshold, Petzke and colleagues[6] performed a series of studies using more sophisticated paradigms that employed random delivery of pressures. These studies showed that (1) the random measures of pressure pain threshold were not influenced by levels of distress of the individual, whereas tender point count and dolorimetry examinations were; (2) fibromyalgia patients were much more sensitive to pressure even when these more sophisticated paradigms were used; (3) fibromyalgia patients were not any more "expectant" or "hypervigilant" than controls; and (4) pressure pain thresholds at any four points in the body are highly correlated with the average tenderness at all 18 tender points and four control points (the thumbnail and forehead).

Responses to other sensory stimuli

Gerster and colleagues[7] were the first to show that fibromyalgia patients also display a low noxious threshold to auditory tones, and this finding was subsequently replicated. However, both of these studies used ascending measures of auditory threshold, so these findings could theoretically be due to expectancy or hypervigilance. A recent study by Geisser and colleagues[8] used an identical random staircase paradigm to test fibromyalgia patients' threshold to the loudness of auditory tones and to pressure. This study found that fibromyalgia patients displayed low thresholds to both types of stimuli, and the correlation between the results of auditory and pressure pain threshold testing suggested that some of this was due to shared variance and some was unique to one stimulus or the other. The notion that fibromyalgia and related syndromes might represent biological amplification of all sensory stimuli has significant support from functional imaging studies that suggest that the insula is the most consistently hyperactive region (see below). This region has been noted to play a critical role in sensory integration, with the posterior insula serving a purer sensory role and the anterior insula being associated with the emotional processing of sensations.[9]

Specific mechanisms that may lead to a low pain threshold in fibromyalgia

Two different pathogenic mechanisms in fibromyalgia have been identified using experimental pain testing: (1) an absence of descending analgesic activity (Fig. 4.2) and (2) increased wind-up or temporal summation.

Attenuated diffuse noxious inhibitory controls in fibromyalgia

In healthy humans and laboratory animals, application of an intense painful stimulus for 2 to 5 minutes produces generalized whole-body analgesia. This analgesic effect, termed *diffuse noxious inhibitory controls* (DNIC), has been consistently observed to be attenuated or absent in groups of fibromyalgia patients compared to healthy controls. The DNIC response in humans is believed to be partly mediated by descending opioidergic pathways and partly by descending serotonergic-noradrenergic pathways. In fibromyalgia, the accumulating data suggest that opioidergic activity is normal or even increased, in that levels of cerebrospinal fluid enkephalins are roughly twice as high in fibromyalgia and idiopathic low back pain

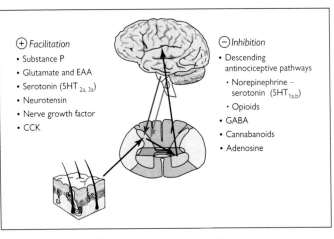

Figure 4.2 Descending influences on nociceptive processing.

patients as in healthy controls. Moreover, positron emission tomography data show that baseline μ opioid receptor binding is decreased in multiple pain-processing regions in the brains of fibromyalgia patients, consistent (but not pathognomonic) with the hypothesis that there is increased release of endogenous μ opioid ligands in fibromyalgia, leading to high baseline occupancy of the receptors.[10] The biochemical and imaging findings suggesting increased activity of endogenous opioidergic systems in fibromyalgia are consistent with the anecdotal experience that opioids are generally ineffective analgesics in patients with fibromyalgia and related conditions. In contrast, studies have shown the opposite for serotonergic and noradrenergic activity in fibromyalgia. Studies have shown that the principal metabolite of norepinephrine, 3-methoxy-4-hydroxyphenethylene (MPHG), is lower in the cerebrospinal fluid of fibromyalgia patients, and nearly any type of compound that simultaneously raises both serotonin and norepinephrine (tricyclic antidepressants, duloxetine, milnacipran, tramadol) has been shown to be efficacious in treating fibromyalgia and related conditions.

Increased wind-up in fibromyalgia

Experimental pain-testing studies have also suggested that some individuals with fibromyalgia may have evidence of wind-up, indicative of evidence of central sensitization (not to be confused with central *sensitivity*, which is a more general phenomenon).[11] In animal models, this finding is associated with excitatory amino acid (e.g., glutamate) and substance P hyperactivity. Four independent studies have shown that patients with fibromyalgia have approximately three-fold higher concentrations of substance P in the cerebrospinal fluid compared with normal controls. Nerve growth factor, which enhances the production of substance P in afferent neurons, is also elevated in the cerebrospinal fluid. Another important neurotransmitter in pain processing, and one that likely plays some role in fibromyalgia, is glutamate. Glutamate is a major excitatory neurotransmitter in the central nervous system, and cerebrospinal fluid levels of glutamate are twice as high in fibromyalgia patients as in controls. Not only are these levels elevated, but a recent study using proton spectroscopy showed that the glutamate levels in the insula in fibromyalgia change in response to changes in both clinical and experimental pain when patients are treated with acupuncture.[12] Furthermore, medications that seem to act by reducing the release of these excitatory neurotransmitters (e.g., pregabalin, gabapentin) also change the response.

Thus, a number of lines of evidence point to the fact that fibromyalgia is a state of heightened pain or sensory processing, and that this might occur because of high levels of neurotransmitters that increase pain transmission and/or low levels of neurotransmitters that decrease pain transmission.

Abnormalities on functional neuroimaging

Functional neural imaging enables investigators to visualize how the brain processes the sensory experience of pain. The primary modes of functional imaging that have been used in fibromyalgia include functional magnetic resonance imaging (fMRI), single photon emission computed tomography (SPECT), positron emission tomography (PET), and proton spectroscopy (H-MRS).

Single photon emission computed tomography (SPECT)

This was the first functional neuroimaging technique to be used in fibromyalgia. The first trial using SPECT imaging in fibromyalgia patients was conducted by Mountz and associates. Their data indicated that both the caudate and the thalamus of fibromyalgia patients had decreased blood flow. Their findings were largely replicated in a second SPECT study by Kwiatek and colleagues.[13] In a third SPECT trial, Guedj and associates[14] used a more sensitive radioligand (99mTc-ECD) in fibromyalgia patients and pain-free controls. They found hyperperfusion in fibromyalgia patients in the somatosensory cortex and hypoperfusion in the anterior and posterior cingulate, the amygdala, the medial frontal and parahippocampal gyrus, and the cerebellum. One longitudinal treatment trial used SPECT imaging to assess changes in regional cerebral blood flow after administration of amitriptyline in 14 fibromyalgia patients. After 3 months of treatment with amitriptyline, increases in blood flow in the bilateral thalamus and the basal ganglia were observed. Since the same two regions had been implicated previously, these data suggest that amitriptyline may normalize the altered blood flow, thereby reducing pain symptoms.

Functional MRI (fMRI)

fMRI is a noninvasive brain imaging technique that relies on changes in the relative concentration of oxygenated to deoxygenated hemoglobin within the brain.

The first study to use fMRI in fibromyalgia patients was performed by Gracely and associates. In this study 16 fibromyalgia patients and 16 matched controls were exposed to painful pressures during the fMRI experiment.[15] The authors found increased neural activations (i.e., increases in the BOLD signal) in patients compared to pain-free controls when stimuli of equal pressure magnitude were administered. Regions of increased activity included the primary and secondary somatosensory cortex, the insula, and the anterior cingulate, all regions commonly observed in fMRI studies of healthy normal subjects during painful stimuli. Interestingly, when the pain-free controls were subjected to pressures that evoked equivalent pain ratings in the fibromyalgia patients, similar activation patterns were observed. These findings were entirely consistent with the "left shift" in stimulus–response function noted with experimental pain testing and suggest that fibromyalgia patients experience an increased gain or "volume setting" in brain sensory processing systems. These findings have now been replicated by three other studies, one of which used heat instead of pressure pain.

Similar to the findings by Gracely and associates, the authors observed significant increases in the pain ratings of patients and augmented pain processing within the contralateral insula. fMRI has also proved useful in determining how comorbid psychological factors influence pain processing in fibromyalgia. For example, a recent study by Giesecke and associates[16] explored the relationship between depression and enhanced evoked pain sensations in 30 patients with fibromyalgia. The authors found that the anterior insula and amygdala activations were correlated with depressive symptoms, consistent with these regions being involved with affective or motivational aspects of pain processing. However, the degree of neuronal activation in areas of the brain thought to be associated with the "sensory" processing of pain (i.e., where the pain is localized and how intense it is) was not associated with levels of depressive symptoms, or the presence or absence of major depression. These data are consistent with a plethora of evidence in the pain field that there are different regions of the brain responsible for pain processing devoted to sensory intensity versus affective aspects of pain sensation, and suggest that the former and latter are largely independent of each other. In contrast, this same group showed that the presence of catastrophizing (a patient's negative or pessimistic appraisal of pain) influences both the sensory and affective dimensions of pain on fMRI in fibromyalgia.

Positron emission tomography

This technique has been used in several studies in fibromyalgia. In the first such study, Yunus and colleagues did not find any differences in regional cerebral blood flow between fibromyalgia patients and controls. However, Wood and colleagues used PET to show that attenuated dopaminergic activity may be playing a role in pain transmission in fibromyalgia, and Harris and colleagues showed evidence of decreased μ opioid receptor availability (possibly due to increased release of endogenous μ opioids) in fibromyalgia.

Other serologic and biochemical abnormalities

Autoantibodies

The search for representative autoantibodies is a predictable step for a disease like fibromyalgia, often evaluated by rheumatologists and coexisting with autoimmune diseases. Antiserotonin antibody, antiganglioside antibody, and antiphospholipid antibody have been shown to be different in patients and controls, but the applicability of these findings is not yet clear. Antiserotonin antibody has been shown to be increased in fibromyalgia in three cross-sectional studies by two different groups. Antiganglioside antibody and antiphospholipid antibody have each been shown to be increased in fibromyalgia in two cross-sectional studies by the same group. A different group evaluating antiganglioside antibody in a third cross-sectional study was unable to reproduce the results. Antithromboplastin antibody, antipolymer antibody, anti-68/84, and anti-45kDa have each been evaluated in one cross-sectional study and have shown increased levels in fibromyalgia. Review of the literature suggests that ANA, antithyroid antibodies, antisilicone antibodies, and anti–glutamic acid decarboxylase are not informative in fibromyalgia.

This inconsistent increase in antibodies to a number of antigens may be a nonspecific finding that arises from a subtle shift in immune function in this spectrum of illness. In the closely related chronic fatigue syndrome and Gulf War illnesses, investigators have noted a shift from a TH1 to a TH2 immune response, which would be expected to lead to increased production of nonspecific antibodies. Thus any antibody or autoantibody proposed as either a diagnostic test or biomarker of fibromyalgia must be carefully tested using stringent controls to ensure its authenticity.

Other biochemical and cytokine abnormalities

The amino acid tryptophan and the cytokine IL-8 have both been shown to be different in patients compared to controls in a couple of studies, but neither has been evaluated in longitudinal studies. Low tryptophan, a precursor for serotonin, has been found in two of three studies by three different groups. IL-8 has been consistently shown in three studies by two different groups. Moreover, IL-8 has been shown to correlate with symptoms and not to be associated with depressed fibromyalgia. IL-8 levels are closely tied to autonomic function, and the findings of these increased levels could be due to the dysautonomia seen in fibromyalgia and related conditions. Glial cells also can produce and modulate cytokines. Their role in fibromyalgia is uncertain.[17]

Structural abnormalities in fibromyalgia

Although a few studies have found mild abnormalities in the skeletal muscles of fibromyalgia patients (these findings have been inconsistent and may be due to deconditioning rather than the illness itself), a few studies suggest there may be subsets of fibromyalgia patients with damage to neural structures. P-31 spectroscopy has been used to examine muscle metabolism in fibromyalgia, and the results are conflicting: one study comparing sedentary controls to fibromyalgia patients found no differences, and the other found lower ATP levels in fibromyalgia patients. Studies suggest that the tenderness in fibromyalgia is not confined to the muscle, so in aggregate most investigators have concluded that primary muscle disease is not a likely cause of the pain associated with fibromyalgia. There are recent data, however, suggesting that a subset of fibromyalgia patients may have abnormalities involving small sensory nerves in the skin, indicative of a small-fiber neuropathy.

There are also emerging data suggesting that there may be subtle abnormalities in brain structure seen in fibromyalgia. Thus, if there are structural abnormalities or damage to tissues in fibromyalgia, the most evidence for this is involving neural tissues.

Sleep and fibromyalgia

In addition to pain, other symptoms commonly seen in fibromyalgia include disturbed sleep and poor physical function. One of the first biological findings in fibromyalgia was that selective sleep deprivation led to symptoms of fibromyalgia in healthy individuals, and these findings have been replicated by several groups.[18] However, the electroencephalographic abnormalities that were noted in this first study and were initially thought to be a marker for fibromyalgia (so-called alpha intrusions) have subsequently been found to be present in normals and in individuals with other conditions. More recent findings on polysomnography that occur more commonly in fibromyalgia include fewer sleep spindles, an increase in cyclic alternating pattern rate, upper airway resistance syndrome, and poor sleep efficiency. However, sleep abnormalities rarely are shown to correlate with symptoms in fibromyalgia, and many investigators anecdotally believe that identifying and treating specific sleep disorders often seen in fibromyalgia patients (e.g., obstructive sleep apnea, upper airway resistance, restless leg or periodic limb movement syndromes) does not necessarily lead to improvements in the core symptoms of fibromyalgia.

Behavioral and psychological factors

In addition to neurobiological mechanisms, behavioral and psychological factors also play a role in symptom expression in many fibromyalgia patients. The rate of current psychiatric comorbidity in patients with FM may be as high as 30% to 60% in tertiary care settings, and the rate of lifetime psychiatric disorders even higher. Depression and anxiety disorders are the most commonly seen. However, these rates may be artifactually elevated by virtue of the fact that most of these studies have been performed in tertiary care centers. Individuals who meet ACR criteria for fibromyalgia who are identified in the general population do not have nearly so high a rate of identifiable psychiatric conditions (Figs. 4.3 and 4.4).

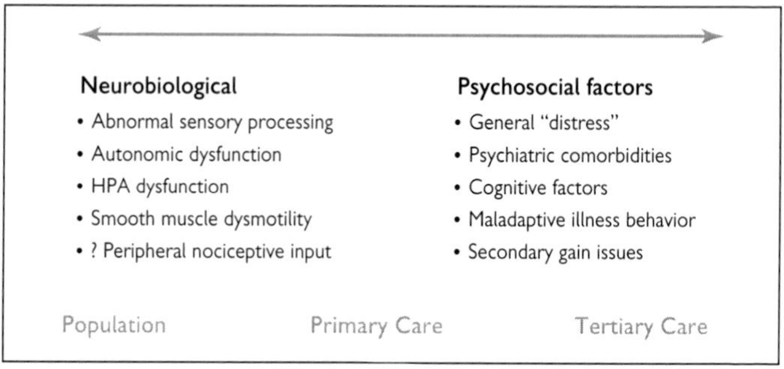

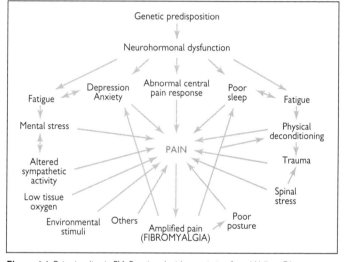

Neurobiological
- Abnormal sensory processing
- Autonomic dysfunction
- HPA dysfunction
- Smooth muscle dysmotility
- ? Peripheral nociceptive input

Psychosocial factors
- General "distress"
- Psychiatric comorbidities
- Cognitive factors
- Maladaptive illness behavior
- Secondary gain issues

Population   Primary Care   Tertiary Care

Figure 4.3 The physiological–psychobehavioral continuum.

Genetic predisposition

Neurohormonal dysfunction

Fatigue

Depression
Anxiety

Abnormal central
pain response

Poor
sleep

Fatigue

Mental stress

Physical
deconditioning

Altered
sympathetic
activity

PAIN

Trauma

Low tissue
oxygen

Spinal
stress

Environmental
stimuli

Others

Amplified pain
(FIBROMYALGIA)

Poor
posture

Figure 4.4 Pain signaling in FM. Reprinted with permission from Wallace DJ. *Fibromyalgia: An Essential Guide for Patients and Their Families.* New York: Oxford University Press.

References

1. Arnold LM, Hudson JI, Hess EV, et al. Family study of fibromyalgia. *Arthritis Rheum.* 2004;50:944–952.

2. Buskila D. Genetics of chronic pain states. *Best Pract Res Clin Rheumatol.* 2007;21:535–547.

3. Sapolsky RM. Why stress is bad for your brain. *Science.* 1996;273:749–750.

4. Crofford LJ, Pillemer SR, Kalogeras KT, et al. Hypothalamic-pituitary-adrenal axis perturbations in patients with fibromyalgia. *Arthritis Rheum.* 1994;37:1583–1592.

5. Martinez-Lavin M, Hermosillo AG, Rosas M, Soto ME. Circadian studies of autonomic nervous balance in patients with fibromyalgia: a heart rate variability analysis. *Arthritis Rheum.* 1998;41:1966–1971.

6. Petzke F, Clauw DJ, Ambrose K, Khine A, Gracely RH. Increased pain sensitivity in fibromyalgia: effects of stimulus type and mode of presentation. *Pain.* 2003;105:403–413.

7. Gerster JC, Hadj-Djilani A. Hearing and vestibular abnormalities in primary fibrositis syndrome. *J Rheumatol.* 1984;11:678–680.

8. Geisser ME, Gracely RH, Giesecke T, et al. The association between experimental and clinical pain measures among persons with fibromyalgia and chronic fatigue syndrome. *Eur J Pain.* 2007;11:202–207.

9. Craig AD. Human feelings: why are some more aware than others? *Trends Cogn Sci.* 2004;8:239–241.

10. Harris RE, Clauw DJ, Scott DJ, et al. Decreased central mu-opioid receptor availability in fibromyalgia. *J Neurosci.* 2007;27:10000–10006.

11. Price DD, Staud D, Robinson ME, et al. Enhanced temporal summation of second pain and its central modulation in fibromyalgia patients. *Pain.* 2002;99:49–59.

12. Harris RE, Sundgren PC, Pang Y, et al. Dynamic levels of glutamate within the insula are associated with improvements in multiple pain domains in fibromyalgia. *Arthritis Rheum.* 2008;58:903–907.

13. Kwiatek R, Barnden L, Rowe C, Pile K. Pontine tegmental regional cerebral blood flow (rCBF) is reduced in fibromyalgia. *Arthritis Rheum.* 1997;40:S43.

14. Guedj E, Taieb D, Cammileri S, et al. 99mTc-ECD brain perfusion SPECT in hyperalgesic fibromyalgia. *Eur J Nucl Med Mol Imaging.* 2007;34:130–134.

15. Gracely RH, Petzke F, Wolf JM, Clauw DJ. Functional magnetic resonance imaging evidence of augmented pain processing in fibromyalgia. *Arthritis Rheum.* 2002;46:1333–1343.

16. Giesecke T, Gracely RH, Williams DA, et al. The relationship between depression, clinical pain, and experimental pain in a chronic pain cohort. *Arthritis Rheum.* 2005;52:1577–1584.

17. Wallace DJ, Linker-Israeli M, Hallegua D, et al. Cytokines play an aetiopathogenetic role in fibromyalgia: a hypothesis and pilot study. *Rheumatology.* 2001;40(7):743–749.

18. Moldofsky H, Scarisbrick P, England R, Smythe H. Musculoskeletal symptoms and non-REM sleep disturbance in patients with "fibrositis syndrome" and healthy subjects. *Psychosom Med.* 1975;37:341–351.

Chapter 5

Clinical findings—symptoms and signs

Patients with fibromyalgia have myriad complaints and a paucity of physical findings other than tender points. This chapter reviews these features[1–5] (Table 5.1).

Table 5.1 Prevalence of symptoms and signs in fibromyalgia patients

Sign/symptom	Prevalence (%)
Widespread pain with tender points	100
Generalized weakness, muscle and joint aches	80
Unrefreshing sleep	75
Fatigue	75
Stiffness	70
Anxiety	60
Psychological stress	60
Dizziness/vertigo	55
Tension headache	55
Cognitive impairment, "fibro-fog"	50
Painful periods	40
Irritable colon	40
Subjective numbness, burning, tingling	35
Subjective complaints of swelling or edema	35
Depression	35
Skin redness, lace-like skin mottling	30
Complaints of fever	20
Complaints of swollen glands	20
Complaints of non-medication dryness, dry eyes	18
Post-traumatic stress disorder	18
Nocturnal myoclonus, restless legs syndrome	15
Raynaud's	15
Irritable bladder, interstitial cystitis	12
Chronic pelvic pain	12
Bipolar illness	10
Reflex sympathetic dystrophy	5

Adapted and updated from Yunus M, Masi AT, Calabro JJ, et al. Primary fibromyalgia (fibrositis): clinical study of 50 patients with matched normal controls. Semin Arthritis Rheum. 1981;11:151–171.

Pain

Because pain is a defining feature of fibromyalgia, it is helpful to focus on the features of the pain that can help distinguish it from other disorders. The pain of fibromyalgia is typically diffuse or multifocal, often waxes and wanes, and is frequently migratory in nature. These characteristics of "central pain" are quite different from "peripheral" pain, where both the location and severity of pain are typically more constant. Patients may complain of discomfort when they are touched or when wearing tight clothing, and they may experience dysesthesias or paresthesias that accompany the pain.

Fatigue

Defined as weariness or physical or mental exhaustion, fatigue is a predominant feature of fibromyalgia. It can be intermittent or continuous. This may occur in parallel with pain and other symptoms (especially cognitive dysfunction) or independently. Emotional stressors, depression, physical illness, difficulty sleeping, poor eating habits, substance abuse, medications, inflammation, hormone imbalances, infections, or cytokine dysregulation could theoretically contribute to fatigue.

Temperature dysregulation

Patients with fibromyalgia often feel feverish or cold (this, like other fibromyalgia symptoms, is a sensory experience) but should not have objective evidence of a fever. Sensory amplification, dysautonomia, or psychiatric disorders might produce this perception. Individuals who complain of fevers should be asked to take their temperature three times daily (morning, midafternoon, and evening) for a week to chart their actual temperatures, as this can be helpful clinically.

Swollen or tender glands

True lymphadenopathy can be part of the initial, transient presentation of postinfectious fibromyalgia but should not be present chronically. In fact, "lymphadenopathy" was eliminated from the definition for chronic fatigue syndrome in 1994, when it was realized that patients with this condition do not have true adenopathy, but instead have the sensation that their lymph nodes are swollen or tender. The presence of allergies, infections, inflammatory processes, anxiety (a form of "globus hystericus"), cancer, or simply body thinness should be assessed.

Myalgias

Muscle aches are common and can occur anywhere but are most often in the upper or lower neck and back. They are usually bilateral and present as a dull, throbbing discomfort. Spasm, defined as an involuntary muscle contraction, is less common than the sense of tightness in muscles that seems like spasm. Muscle aches may worsen after exercise or activity. They tend to be worse in the late afternoon and early evening and to feel "flu-like." Although patients complain of weakness or lack of endurance, muscle strength is typically normal on physical examination unless the patient has become very sedentary and deconditioned. Reports have suggested that muscle weakness or fatigue is a feature of fibromyalgia, but it is difficult to discriminate this from a deconditioned state since fibromyalgia patients may feel worse with exercise and tend to avoid it.

Arthralgias

Joints are not objectively swollen or inflamed in fibromyalgia unless the individual has concomitant arthritis (and this is common). Nonetheless, patients with fibromyalgia often have this complaint, perhaps because of the overall sensory hypersensitivity they experience. Fibromyalgia tender points such as the anserine bursa of the knee or lateral epicondyle can also convey a sensation of joint aching, as can cutaneous hyperesthesia overlying joints.

Stiffness

A gel-like sensation, or stiffness, is very common and widespread in fibromyalgia. It may be present in the morning but often worsens in the later afternoon or early evening, and can be particularly troublesome when the afflicted individual is sitting or staying in any position for a prolonged period. Stiffness may be aggravated by changes in barometric pressure, poor sleep, anxiety, stress, or physical activity. Relieving factors include local heat, moderate activities, massage, or stretching exercises. Pain and stiffness strongly correlate with each other.

Soft tissue discomfort and nodularity

Soft tissues include the supporting structures of joints such as tendons, bursae, and ligaments, as well as the myofascia. The myofascia lies between the dermis and muscles and consists of connective tissue and fat, which buffer muscles and provide structural integrity and support. The ACR tender points represent the most frequent areas of myofascial discomfort. The presence of "nodules" may be common in some of the upper back and lower neck regions. They tend to be firm, mobile, globular or spindle-shaped tender structures consisting of fatty tissue, fibrous cords, and muscles. Inflammation is not present.

Hypermobility

Some reports suggest an association between benign hypermobility syndrome and fibromyalgia.

Neurologic manifestations

Headache: Tension and migraine

Both tension and migraine headaches are strongly linked with fibromyalgia, especially tension headache, which may simply represent a form of myofascial pain involving the head. A sustained muscular contraction in the forehead, jaw, or temporal areas can produce headache-like pain, frequently described as a dull, tight band around the head. These are muscular contraction headaches and are not truly neurologic in nature. Occipital tender points with or without cervical osteoarthritis are associated with headaches emanating from the back of the head. Vasomotor instability is a manifestation of autonomic dysfunction, a feature that is prevalent in fibromyalgia. When unilateral and associated with photophobia, pounding, and a premonitory aura, it often represents a form of migraine. Medication-related headaches, sinus headaches, and osteoarthritis-related headaches should be ruled out.

Cognitive dysfunction

The term *fibro-fog* has been used to describe the fact that fibromyalgia patients have difficulty remembering names and dates, balancing their checkbook, or focusing. Common complaints are confusion, memory blanks, word mix-ups, altered information processing, and concentration difficulties. These symptoms can be fleeting or intermittent but are rarely constant (which differentiates it from dementias) and are worsened by anxiety or stress. Although self-report of cognitive impairment is common, it is less commonly noted by observers, and intellectual capacity is usually normal.

Numbness, burning, and tingling

These symptoms may be reported in any part of the body (they rarely follow a single dermatome) and tend to come and go. They have been described as a "pins and needles" sensation and can have a radiating quality. Physical findings and neurologic examination are usually normal, as are nerve biopsies and electrical testing with electromyography and nerve conduction velocities. Many patients have had unnecessary carpal tunnel surgeries and other procedures for these complaints. In fact, painful nerve sensations are a mild form of local nerve compression caused by autonomic dysfunction (see the later section on swelling) or altered sensory perception due to central sensitization. True radiculopathy, spinal stenosis or Chiari malformation, or other neurologic disorders should be considered in the differential diagnosis.

Insomnia

Most fibromyalgia patients have some difficulty with sleep, ranging from difficulty falling asleep to difficulty staying asleep, or at a minimum report awakening in the morning not feeling refreshed. Although some fibromyalgia patients have sleep apnea or hypopnea, it is probable that upper-airway resistance syndrome or periodic leg movements may play a more significant role in those with fibromyalgia and with altered sleep architecture.

Comorbidities such as cardiopulmonary disease, smoking, coughing, allergies, or the use of caffeine or alcohol may worsen these problems.

Restless legs syndrome

Restless legs syndrome may be present in up to 10% of the U.S. population but has been reported in 20% to 50% of those with fibromyalgia. Restless legs syndrome is a form of periodic limb movement syndrome also known as sleep myoclonus; patients complain of a sudden jerking, lifting, shooting out, or movement in their legs during sleep. Individuals are often alerted to this sleep behavior by their bed partners. Patients can feel a need to move their legs, which is relieved by moving or walking. Manifested electrically as an alpha-wave burst followed by limb movement, restless leg syndrome is found in individuals who have excess sympathetic tone, possible iron deficiency, and hypoxia, as well as more movement arousals and less stage 3 and 4 sleep. These patients are less responsive to usually prescribed sleep medications but often do well with dopaminergic agonists. This may represent a subset of fibromyalgia patients who might be more likely to respond to dopamine agonists.

Bruxism

Temporomandibular joint dysfunction syndrome is a regional manifestation of myofascial discomfort that is also a feature of fibromyalgia. Most of these patients grind their teeth, and bruxism is a manifestation of this syndrome associated with compromised sleep. This is sometimes improved with the use of night splints.

Neuro-otologic symptoms

Patients report dry and irritated eyes and dry mouth, and some have mild objective evidence of this on formal testing, accounting for a large overlap between fibromyalgia and Sjögren syndrome. Although aggravated by drying medications (especially tricyclic antidepressants), some individuals are not taking any of these agents. Light-headedness, dizziness, or sensitivity to bright lights or loud noises likely represents a global sensory hyperactivity. Some patients have had syncopal reactions and dizziness, again perhaps in part due to the known overlap with neurally mediated hypotension and postural orthostatic tachycardia.

Cardiovascular and chest complaints

A variety of thoracic symptoms are frequently noted in fibromyalgia. These include costochondritis (Tietze syndrome), which is inclusive of an ACR tender point; palpitations (presumably due to dysautonomia and/or sensory hypersensitivity); noncardiac chest pain; and gastroesophageal reflux. There is a subset of individuals with persistent low blood pressure who have neurally mediated hypotension. This may be noted in 10% to 20% of patients with fibromyalgia; it is clinically associated with fatigue and feeling faint. Impaired variability of the R-R interval on electrocardiography (i.e., heart rate variability) is a dysautonomic feature of fibromyalgia.

Swelling

Over one-third of patients with fibromyalgia are bothered by a sensation of fluid retention, or edema. Physical examination rarely demonstrates evidence of swelling, and diuretics are typically only transiently beneficial.

Cutaneous and cutaneovascular findings

Dry skin, hair loss, and itching are more common complaints in fibromyalgia than in controls. The presence of a lace-like, checkerboard red/white skin mottling known as livedo reticularis is statistically associated with fibromyalgia but is almost always asymptomatic. This likely occurs because of disordered autonomically mediated flow to the subpapillary and dermal blood vessels. True Raynaud's phenomenon is not known to occur more commonly with fibromyalgia, but patients often have color changes in their hands or feet. In contrast to true Raynaud's, in fibromyalgia there is not a clear demarcation between affected and unaffected areas, nor is there the classic triphasic color change. Some of these patients are misdiagnosed as having an autoimmune disorder, especially when they present with low-titer, nonspecific autoantibodies.

Endocrine abnormalities

Sex hormone imbalance may aggravate or ameliorate fibromyalgia symptoms. Females with fibromyalgia tend to have lower androgen levels than age-matched controls. Several studies have suggested that elevated prolactin levels, decreased nocturnal growth hormone secretion, and mild hypocortisolemia with increased corticotropin-releasing hormone responsiveness may be a feature of fibromyalgia. Thyroid does not appear to play an etiopathogenic role. The clinical implications of these subtle abnormalities are not clear.

Dysautonomias

The autonomic nervous system includes our "fight-or-flight" mechanism and regulates pulse and blood pressure with vasomotor adjustments in vascular tone. It also mediates muscular contraction, sweat, urine, and defecation reflexes. Fibromyalgia is associated with a dysregulated autonomic nervous system, primarily involving the sympathetic nervous system.[4] Epinephrine, norepinephrine, dopamine, and acetylcholine help transmit autonomic instructions via the descending nerve tracts. This dysregulation might lead to sympathetic mediated pain and perhaps the clinical manifestations listed in Table 5.2. Parasympathetic dysfunction plays a major role with irritable bowel syndrome. Sustained, unopposed stimulation of the sympathetic nervous system can lead to neurogenic inflammation and reflex sympathetic dystrophy (complex regional pain syndrome type I) (see Chapter 7).

Table 5.2 Symptoms and signs of fibromyalgia where sympathetic tone *may* play a role

- Cardiovascular: neurally mediated hypotension, mitral valve prolapse, palpitations, swelling
- Cutaneovascular: Raynaud's, livedo reticularis
- Neurologic: cognitive dysfunction, paresthesias, vascular headaches
- Neuro-otologic: dizziness, dry eyes and mouth
- Generalized hypervigilance
- Reflex sympathetic dystrophy (complex regional pain syndrome, type 1)

Psychological, behavioral, and cognitive factors

In addition to neurobiological mechanisms, behavioral and psychological factors also play a role in symptom expression in many fibromyalgia patients. The rate of current psychiatric comorbidity in patients with fibromyalgia may be as high as 30% to 60% in tertiary care settings, and the rate of lifetime psychiatric disorders even higher. Depression and anxiety disorders are the most commonly seen. However, these rates may be artifactually elevated by virtue of the fact that most of these studies have been performed in tertiary care centers. Individuals who meet ACR criteria for fibromyalgia who are identified in the general population do not have nearly so high a rate of identifiable psychiatric conditions.

Other psychiatric conditions such as PTSD and bipolar disorder have been more recently linked with fibromyalgia. PTSD is brought on by a traumatic event or continuous unpleasant circumstances. More prevalent in patients who have a family history of abuse (sexual, physical, or verbal), domestic violence, alcoholism, or addiction, PTSD is associated with nightmares, recurrent and intensive recollections, hypervigilance, fear, catastrophizing, and avoidance of thoughts associated with the event. PTSD is also more prevalent in individuals who served in the military and saw action. Familial studies have also shown that patients with bipolar illness are at a 150-fold increased risk for developing fibromyalgia. Bipolar illness affects 1% of the U.S. population but may be present in up to 10% of fibromyalgia patients. Its treatment is particularly frustrating, as these patients respond poorly to musculoskeletal and pain-directed interventions.

As already noted, population-based studies have shown that the relationship between pain and distress is complex and that distress is both a cause and a consequence of pain. In the latter instance, a typical pattern is that as a result of pain and other symptoms of fibromyalgia, individuals begin to function less well in their various roles. They may have difficulties with spouses, children, and work inside or outside the home, which exacerbates symptoms and leads to maladaptive illness behaviors. These include isolation, cessation of pleasurable activities, reductions in activity and exercise, and so forth. In the worst cases, patients become involved with disability and compensation systems. This almost ensures that they will not improve.

The complex interaction of biological, behavioral, and psychological mechanisms is not, however, unique to fibromyalgia. Nonbiological factors play a prominent role in symptom expression in all rheumatic diseases. In fact, in conditions such as rheumatoid arthritis and osteoarthritis, non-biological factors such as level of formal education, coping strategies, and socioeconomic variables account for more of the variance in pain report and disability than biologic factors such as the joint space width or sedimentation rate.

Unique features in certain fibromyalgia populations

Males with fibromyalgia

Males represent only 10% of patients with fibromyalgia. Interestingly, they tend to have more severe symptoms, poorer physical functioning, and a lower quality of life than women with fibromyalgia.

Fibromyalgia in the elderly

Patients with fibromyalgia that develops at over 65 years of age represent less than 10% of cases. Much of the time, the development of rheumatoid arthritis, hypothyroidism, polymyalgia rheumatica, diffuse osteoarthritis, or primary Sjögren syndrome can explain new musculoskeletal complaints in this age group. Evaluations of older-onset patients reveal fewer functional symptoms such as anxiety, stress, or unrefreshing sleep but more musculoskeletal complaints than in their younger counterparts.

Fibromyalgia in children and adolescents

Fibromyalgia is less common in children and adolescents than in adults.[5] It is the 12th most common reason for visiting a pediatric rheumatologist, as opposed to the second or third most common reason for consulting an adult rheumatologist. It is also possible that "growing pains" are a *form fruste* of fibromyalgia. Most cases occur in adolescents.

Pediatric rheumatologists are aware that these processes are much more likely to be self-limited and not be chronic in adolescents, in contrast to adults. Given such, they advise against home schooling, which may worsen the condition, and the use of medications is minimized but not avoided. A vigorous exercise program, cognitive-behavioral therapy, biofeedback, physical therapy, and local injections (if needed) are often associated with the best outcomes.

Fibromyalgia and pregnancy

There is no contraindication to becoming pregnant with fibromyalgia, and the syndrome does not affect fertility. Some patients worry about their ability to carry their baby and sleep at night. The major issues with pregnancy and breastfeeding relate to whether medications can be taken or should be discontinued. One study suggested that 25% of patients have flares during gestation, which raises additional concerns relating to introducing medication. These circumstances should be handled on an individual basis, and although not contraindicated, most psychotropic medications, nonsteroidal anti-inflammatories, and muscle relaxants can be taken with close follow-up.

References

1. Wallace DJ, Clauw DJ, Hallegua DS. Addressing behavioral abnormalities in fibromyalgia. *J Musculoskel Med.* 2005;22:562–579.

2. Moldofsky H. Sleep, neuroimmune and neuroendocrine functions in fibromyalgia and chronic fatigue syndrome. *Adv Neuroimmunol.* 1995;5:39–56.

3. Yunus M, Masi AT, Calabro JJ, et al. Primary fibromyalgia (fibrositis): clinical study of 50 patients with matched normal controls. *Semin Arthritis Rheum.* 1981;11:151–171.

4. Martinez-Lavin M, Hermosillo AG. Autonomic nervous system dysfunction may explain the multisystem features of fibromyalgia. *Semin Arthritis Rheum.* 2000;29:197–199.

5. Sherry DD, Malleson PN. The idiopathic musculoskeletal syndromes in childhood, *Rheum Dis Clin North Am.* 2002;28:669–685.

Chapter 6

Laboratory and imaging correlates

The evaluation of an individual with chronic pain is a complex process. In contrast to most other medical problems, simply arriving at a "diagnosis" is typically insufficient to guide treatment. This is because within any given pain diagnosis, there is tremendous heterogeneity with respect to the underlying causes and contributors to symptoms, as well as to the most effective treatments. In particular, individuals with chronic pain can have greater or lesser peripheral nociceptive (i.e., tissue damage, inflammation) and central non-nociceptive (i.e., pain or sensory amplification, psychological factors) contributions to their pain. Therefore, the differential diagnosis of chronic pain involves identifying which of these factors are present in which individuals, so that the appropriate pharmacologic, procedural, and psychological therapies can be administered.

A careful musculoskeletal history and examination remains the most important diagnostic test for musculoskeletal pain. In other fields of medicine, advances in diagnostic testing have rendered a physical examination largely obsolete. However, in musculoskeletal medicine, technology confuses as much as it helps. For example, many healthy, asymptomatic people test positive for antinuclear antibody or rheumatoid factor, or have abnormal results on imaging studies. Worse yet, these diagnostic tests rarely tell us how "severe" the pain is, because there is typically a significant discordance between the results of laboratory or imaging studies and the severity of pain and other symptoms that the individual is experiencing. Therefore, the musculoskeletal history and examination must allow the clinician to arrive at the diagnosis (or at worst a very narrow differential diagnosis). Then, if necessary, further diagnostic testing should be used to confirm these findings.

The clinical laboratory is not helpful in fibromyalgia. However, since fibromyalgia is a diagnosis of exclusion, a routine blood chemistry panel, complete blood count, thyroid blood panel, muscle enzymes, urinalysis, and, if appropriate, autoimmune blood testing should be obtained. Many fibromyalgia patients have low titers of autoantibodies such as rheumatoid factor or antinuclear antibody and are misdiagnosed as having an inflammatory process. If necessary, a bone scan or magnetic resonance imaging can determine whether inflammation is present. Obtaining immune function testing, cytokine levels, or trace elements is not supported by a review of the evidence-based literature. If indicated, a chest radiograph or electrocardiogram may be useful in assessing cardiovascular or chest complaints. Electrical studies such as an electromyogram or nerve conduction velocities may rule out a true radiculopathy or compressive neuropathy. In an investigational setting, elevated spinal fluid levels of nerve growth factor, substance P, or biogenic amines may be associated with fibromyalgia. Most of this information has been derived from functional brain imaging, reviewed in Chapters 4 and 7. Essentially, chronic pain states are associated with reduced isotope blood flow, while acute pain is associated with increased blood flow.

Chapter 7

Clinical associations and subsets

Because symptoms can present in any region of the body, patients with fibromyalgia have often consulted other specialists and received other diagnoses. Some of these diagnoses are in fact other central sensitivity syndromes, whereas others do not exist. Also, additional disorders mimic fibromyalgia. This chapter reviews these considerations.

Clinical associations

Chronic fatigue syndrome (CFS)

The concept of CFS originally evolved as a postinfectious fatigue condition.[1] Intended to encompass profound fatigue in individuals without any psychiatric disorder, the syndrome displays a substantial overlap with fibromyalgia. Many patients diagnosed with CFS demonstrate an abrupt onset of symptoms, temporally related to a presumed or documented infection. Widespread chronic musculoskeletal pain is evident in some, but sometimes individuals have regional pain (e.g., in the muscles, joints, lymph nodes, head) instead. Approximately half of fibromyalgia patients will also meet criteria for CFS (Tables 7.1 and 7.2).

Table 7.1 Centers for Disease Control Revised Criteria for Chronic Fatigue Syndrome (1994)

1. Chronic fatigue of unknown cause that persists or returns for more than 6 months, resulting in a substantial reduction in occupational, educational, social, or personal activities

2. The presence of 4 or more of the following symptoms concurrently for more than 6 months:

    i. sore throat

    ii. tender cervical or axillary lymph glands

    iii. muscle pain

    iv. multijoint pain

    v. new headaches

    vi. unrefreshing sleep

    vii. postexertion malaise

    viii. cognitive dysfunction

Table 7.2 Chronic fatigue syndrome and fibromyalgia: Similarities and differences

Parameter	Fibromyalgia (%)	Chronic fatigue syndrome (%)
Female sex	90	80
Muscle aches	99	80
Joint aches	99	75
Fatigue	80	100
Poor sleep	80	50
Complaints of fever	28	75
Complaints of swollen glands	33	80
Postexertional fatigue	80	80
Sudden or acute onset	55	70
Headaches	60	85
Cognitive dysfunction	20	65

Functional bowel disorders

Functional bowel disorders encompass a variety of diagnostic labels, including irritable bowel syndrome (sometimes referred to as spastic colitis or irritable colon), noncardiac chest pain, non-ulcer dyspepsia, and diffuse abdominal pain.[2] These conditions have all been shown to have underlying abnormalities in pain processing (i.e., visceral and somatic hyperalgesia) as a primary pathophysiologic problem, although other theories, such as those involving motility or bacterial overgrowth, also play a role in subsets of individuals with these conditions. Of patients with these conditions, 70% are females, and the major complaints are distention; bloating, pain relief with bowel movements, more frequent and loose stools with the onset of pain, mucus-containing stools, a sensation of incomplete evacuation, flatulence, or cramping. Celiac disease, medication side effects, small intestinal bacterial overgrowth, and inflammatory bowel conditions should be ruled out (Table 7.3).

Chronic pelvic pain syndromes

The urethra, bladder neck, vagina, and rectum are visceral structures attached to striated (voluntary) muscles. Visceral receptors are usually silent but can cause chronic pain when abnormally activated.

Irritable bladder syndromes

Many patients suffer from urinary urgency or frequency, accompanied by bladder or suprapubic pain. Once infection, malignancy, or other conditions have been excluded, these patients are often diagnosed with interstitial cystitis, painful bladder syndrome, chronic prostatitis, or irritable bladder. These conditions have all been shown to be more prevalent in fibromyalgia patients, and patients with interstitial cystitis or painful bladder syndrome are much more likely to have fibromyalgia.

Table 7.3 Spectrum of functional gastrointestinal disorders

- Esophageal—functional chest pain, heartburn, dysphagia
- Gastroduodenal—dyspepsia (functional, ulcer-like, dysmotility-like), aerophagia, functional vomiting
- Bowel—irritable bowel syndrome (IBS), functional abdominal bloating, constipation, or diarrhea
- Functional abdominal pain
- Functional biliary tract disorders—gallbladder or sphincter of Oddi dysfunction
- Anorectal—anorectal pain, fecal incontinence, proctalgia fugax, pelvic floor dyssynergia

The female pelvic region: "Chronic pelvic congestion"

Pelvic pain can be hormonal, structural, or related to spasm. The release of prostaglandins and other chemicals prior to menses produces fluid retention, bloating, and alterations in mood and behavior and can lead to painful periods (dysmenorrhea). Surveys have suggested that 3% to 10% of menstruating females in the United States have severe physical or psychological symptoms that interfere with their ability to function. Usually manifested premenstrually, these include irritability, tension, headache, backache, breast tenderness, depression, lack of energy, difficulty concentrating or sleeping, and feeling "out of control." Hormonal interventions, mild diuresis, and nonsteroidal anti-inflammatory agents are useful. Selective serotonin reuptake inhibitors such as fluoxetine may be ameliorative as well. Seventy percent of menstruating fibromyalgia patients report premenstrual flares of their symptoms.

Structural causes of chronic pelvic discomfort may or may not be associated with fibromyalgia. These include pelvic inflammatory disease, adenomyosis, leiomyomata, uterine prolapse, ovarian cysts or masses, cervical stenosis, and pelvic adhesions. Conflicting data have been published relating to an association between endometriosis and fibromyalgia.

A small group of fibromyalgia patients describe intense female genital tract discomfort, painful vulva without infection (vulvodynia), or involuntary spasm of the vaginal muscles when intercourse is attempted (vaginismus) or during a normal gynecologic exam. These complaints, which lead to 2% of all gynecology visits in the United States, are statistically associated with irritable bladder complaints. The patient's psychosocial background may include a combination of behaviors or experiences including abuse, domestic violence, a family history of alcoholism, a rape experience, traumatic toilet training, abnormal bowel habits, dance training, pelvic trauma, pelvic inflammatory disease, and guilt surrounding sexual feelings. Repetitive minor trauma or straining at dance, gymnastics, and bicycling or certain other vigorous exercises also play a role. Treatments include counseling, anxiety reduction measures, psychotropic medications, sex therapy, and pelvic floor musculature biofeedback.

Complex regional pain syndrome, type 1

Also known as reflex sympathetic dystrophy (RSD), this is an extreme form of altered sympathetically mediated pain,[3] usually induced by trauma, surgery, or certain drugs. Patients develop burning, tingling or throbbing, sensitivity to touch or cold, and swelling of the arms or legs. It has a prevalence of 1 person per 5000 in the United States. Skin in the affected regions is red or mottled, and the painful extremity is warm, painful to touch, and difficult to move. Eventually the edema gives way to a cold region with atrophy. Most patients with RSD fulfill criteria for fibromyalgia as well. It is a type of causalgia, or sustained burning pain with allodynia, increased reactions to stimuli, and dysautonomia with increased flow to the region (Fig. 7.1). Recent-onset RSD can be diagnosed with three-phase blood-pool nuclear scintigraphy showing increased flow on early images. Early

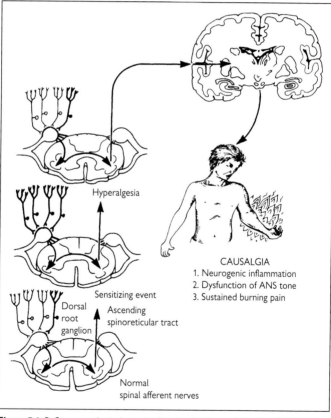

Hyperalgesia

CAUSALGIA
1. Neurogenic inflammation
2. Dysfunction of ANS tone
3. Sustained burning pain

Sensitizing event

Dorsal root ganglion

Ascending spinoreticular tract

Normal spinal afferent nerves

Figure 7.1 Reflex sympathetic dystrophy. Reprinted with permission from Wallace DJ. *Fibromyalgia: An Essential Guide for Patients and Their Families.* New York: Oxford University Press.

RSD is often treated with corticosteroids, vigorous mobilization, physical therapy, and sympathetic blockade.

Autoimmune disorders

Anywhere from 10% to 30% of patients with primary Sjögren syndrome, systemic lupus erythematosus, Hashimoto's thyroiditis, or rheumatoid arthritis also have fibromyalgia. The reasons include untreated or under-treated inflammation (leading to central sensitization or other central pain-amplification mechanisms), hyperesthesia produced by steroids, or steroid withdrawal syndromes. Patients with autoimmune conditions commonly have disease-related psychosocial distress and difficulty coping, which can produce or aggravate fibromyalgia. It can be difficult to distinguish fibromyalgia from autoimmune complaints; the presence of acute-phase reactants supports the latter. Patients with fibromyalgia are also often misdiagnosed as having an autoimmune disorder.

Lyme disease

Patients with documented Lyme disease sometimes have fibromyalgia triggered by their initial infection. A major clinical challenge relates to the debate as to whether there is an entity known as "chronic Lyme" disease (probably not—but how long individuals who remain symptomatic should receive antibiotics is an unanswered question).

Gulf War illnesses

Approximately 70,000 of the 700,000 U.S. men and women who served in the 1991 Persian Gulf War recorded complaints of fatigue (61%), nasal sinus congestion (51%), diarrhea (44%), joint stiffness (41%), irritable colon (41%), myalgias (41%), cognitive impairment (41%), and headache (39%). When strict criteria were applied (symptoms starting 2 to 3 months after leaving the Persian Gulf with a duration of symptoms for 6 months, other diseases having been ruled out), a much higher than expected proportion were shown to have fibromyalgia, chronic fatigue syndrome, irritable bowel syndrome, and many of the other conditions within this spectrum compared to individuals who were in the military but who were not deployed. Similar syndromes have been shown to occur after other wars.

Steroid, alcohol, heroin, or cocaine withdrawal

Individuals exposed to these substances are more hypervigilant and have an increased prevalence of hyperesthesia, especially with chronic corticosteroid administration. Small alterations in steroid dosing can also aggravate fibromyalgia symptoms. Withdrawal from alcohol, heroin, or cocaine producing fibromyalgia-related complaints is usually a self-limited process.

Regional myofascial pain

Also known as *myofascial pain syndrome*, regional myofascial pain is defined as one- to three-quadrant fibromyalgia. More frequent among males than fibromyalgia, it is usually brought on by localized trauma, overuse, or postural abnormalities (e.g., scoliosis). Sustained altered body mechanics result in sensitization of a primary nociceptor and subsequent regional hyperalgesia, allodynia, and referred pain (see Chapter 4). Tender points are common. These are hyperirritable loci found at musculotendinous junctions near nerves where mechanical forces cause microinjuries, and altered central nociception around them leads to enlarged receptor fields and referred pain.

Myofascial pain syndrome can occur anywhere in the body, but five regional combinations account for 90% of all cases: temporomandibular joint dysfunction; neck and upper torso; neck, arm, and hand; low back, buttock, and leg; and the chest area, including costochondritis (Fig. 7.2). Most patients do not have constitutional symptoms associated with fibromyalgia such as fatigue or difficulty concentrating. Jaw pain can be caused by malocclusion, rheumatoid arthritis, trauma, osteoarthritis, or infection. Temporomandibular joint dysfunction is a diagnosis of exclusion that is often seen in patients with chronic widespread pain, anxiety, and teeth grinding (bruxism). Three-quarters of patients with fibromyalgia have temporomandibular-related complaints, but only18% with temporomandibular joint dysfunction meet the criteria for fibromyalgia. Optimal

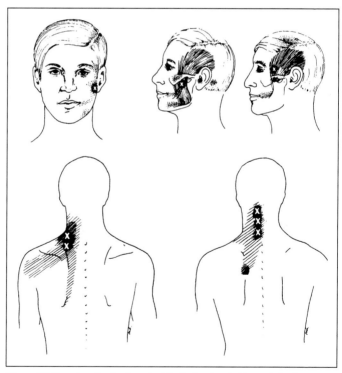

Figure 7.2 Examples of regional myofascial pain. Reprinted with permission from Wallace DJ. *Fibromyalgia: An Essential Guide for Patients and Their Families.* New York: Oxford University Press.

therapy for myofascial pain includes nonsteroidal anti-inflammatories, non-narcotic analgesics, muscle relaxants, moist heat, joint spacers or bite plates worn at night (for temporomandibular joint dysfunction), local applications, injections, exercises, and/or acupuncture. Surgery is rarely beneficial. Ergonomic evaluations of workstations can identify regions of repetitive strains, and physical or occupational therapy may be helpful. Untreated regional myofascial pain can lead to more widespread pain and full-blown fibromyalgia.

Subgroups of fibromyalgia patients

Because of the biopsychosocial nature of fibromyalgia, several groups have attempted to identify subgroups of individuals with this condition, which may present differently or respond differently to treatment.[4] One of these studies examined how differential degrees of depression, maladaptive cognitions, and hyperalgesia might interact to lead to different subgroups of patients.

Three identified subgroups can be usefully identified (Fig. 7.3). The first represents approximately half of the patients who have low levels of depression and anxiety and normal cognition regarding pain and are mildly tender (although tender enough to meet the ACR criteria). The

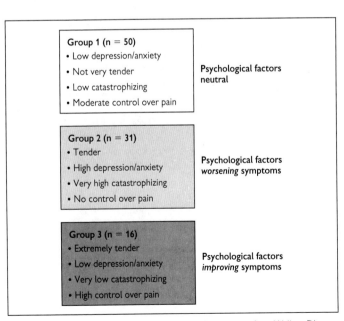

Figure 7.3 Subgroups of FM Patients. Reprinted with permission from Wallace DJ. *Fibromyalgia: An Essential Guide for Patients and Their Families.* New York: Oxford University Press.

second subgroup, representative of a "tertiary care" fibromyalgia patient, is slightly more tender and also displays high levels of depression. These patients also have cognitions associated with a poor prognosis in many pain conditions. These include an external locus of pain control, defined as feeling that they can do nothing about their pain, and catastrophizing, defined as having a very negative and pessimistic view of their pain. The third subgroup, and perhaps the most interesting, is the most tender but has no negative psychological or cognitive factors. This suggests that in some "resilient" individuals, positive psychological and cognitive factors may actually buffer neurobiological factors leading to pain and other symptoms in fibromyalgia.

Use of functional imaging in fibromyalgia

Functional imaging studies have been instructive with regard to how these comorbid mood disorders or cognitions may be influencing pain processing in fibromyalgia. Functional MRI in 30 fibromyalgia patients with variable levels of depression, with additional experimental pain testing, was done to investigate how the presence or absence of depression influences pain report.[3] This study found that the level of depressive symptomatology did not influence the degree of neuronal activation in brain regions responsible for coding for the sensory intensity of pain, the primary and secondary somatosensory cortices. As expected, the depressed individuals displayed greater activations in brain regions known to be responsible for the affective or cognitive processing of pain, such as the amygdala and insula. Another study with similar methodology examined how the presence or absence of catastrophizing might influence pain report in fibromyalgia. In contrast to the results above, the presence of catastrophizing was associated with increased neuronal activations in the sensory coding regions. These studies thus provide empirical evidence for the value of treatments such as cognitive-behavioral therapy. This is especially true if individuals exhibit cognitions such as catastrophizing, which, independent of other factors, may be capable of increasing pain intensity.

References

1. Campbell SM. Regional myofascial pain syndromes. *Rheum Dis Clin North Am.* 1989;15:31–44.

2. Fukuda K, Straus SE, Hickie I, et al., International Chronic Fatigue Study Group. The chronic fatigue syndrome: a comprehensive approach to its definition and study. *Ann Intern Med.* 1999;308:763–766.

3. Giesecke T, Gracely RH, Williams DA, et al. The relationship between depression, clinical pain, and experimental pain in a chronic pain cohort. *Arthritis Rheum.* 2005;52:1577–1584

4. Giesecke T, Williams DA, Harris RE, et al. Subgrouping of fibromyalgia patients on the basis of pressure-pain thresholds and psychological factors. *Arthritis Rheum.* 2003;48:2916–2922.

Chapter 8

Differential diagnosis

Individuals with vague or diffuse complaints are all too often dismissed as having fibromyalgia. In turn, they may advertise the diagnosis to physicians, family, and friends. All too often, this results in "pigeonholing," whereby other comorbidities, conditions, or diagnoses are not considered or treated. Fibromyalgia can be diagnosed only after other conditions are excluded, and the blood tests and imaging and electrical studies that can be helpful in the diagnosis are reviewed in Chapter 6.

Is it really fibromyalgia?

Many common conditions can simulate fibromyalgia or coexist with it.[1] These are summarized in Table 8.1.

Hormonal imbalances

Hypothyroid patients are frequently tired and achy but are readily identified by an elevated circulating thyroid stimulating hormone level. Hyperparathyroidism and hypercalcemia cause aching, weakness, and musculoskeletal pain. An increased percentage of patients with fibromyalgia or other types of chronic pain are deficient in vitamin D, but no studies have yet determined whether replacing vitamin D in this setting reduces pain in these individuals. Patients with an early pregnancy, recent-onset diabetes, and evolving menopause have all been misdiagnosed as having fibromyalgia due to overlapping symptoms. Low cortisol levels in adrenally deficient patients produce profound fatigue, electrolyte imbalances, and aching.

Infections

Microbes infecting the body induce a variety of systemic reactions, including fatigue, malaise, fever, adenopathy, rashes, arthralgias, shortness of breath, abdominal pain, and cognitive dysfunction. Infections can aggravate a pre-existing fibromyalgia, trigger a postinfectious fibromyalgia, or be mistaken for fibromyalgia.

Musculoskeletal and gastrointestinal disorders

Fibromyalgia is a noninflammatory syndrome. Rheumatoid arthritis, systemic lupus erythematosus, Sjögren syndrome, spondyloarthropathies, palindromic rheumatism, and polymyalgia rheumatica are inflammatory disorders. In other words, patients with these disorders typically have elevated acute-phase reactants (e.g., sedimentation rate, C-reactive protein,

Table 8.1 Common conditions that should be differentiated from fibromyalgia

1. Hormone imbalances
   - Menstrual disorders
   - Hypothyroidism
   - Low vitamin D
   - Hyperparathyroidism
   - Pregnancy
   - Adrenal insufficiency
   - Early diabetes
   - Menopause
2. Infections
   - Bacteria
   - Viruses
   - Fungi
   - Parasites
3. Musculoskeletal and autoimmune disorders
   - Rheumatoid arthritis
   - Seronegative spondyloarthropathies in females
   - Lyme disease
   - Lupus
   - Palindromic rheumatism
   - Inflammatory bowel disease prodromes
   - Celiac disease
   - Polymyalgia rheumatica
   - Primary Sjögren syndrome
4. Neurologic disease
   - Multiple sclerosis
   - Myasthenia gravis
5. Malignancy
6. Substance abuse
7. Malnutrition
8. Primary psychiatric disorders
9. Allergies

low complements) or positive serologies (e.g., elevated anti-DNA, anti-CCP), an abnormal protein electrophoresis (e.g., polyclonal gammopathy, elevated alpha-1 or -2 globulins), or evidence of synovitis on imaging.

The problem lies with patients who have both an inflammatory disorder and fibromyalgia (20% to 30%), those with a reaction to an anti-inflammatory drug that leads to myofascial pain (e.g., corticosteroids, interferons), or those misdiagnosed with an inflammatory process who in fact have only fibromyalgia. Spondyloarthropathies are statistically associated with inflammatory bowel disorders, and women with this disorder have a more subtle presentation that can be misdiagnosed as fibromyalgia. Also, celiac disease and small intestinal bacterial overgrowth may be mistakenly diagnosed as functional bowel disorders.

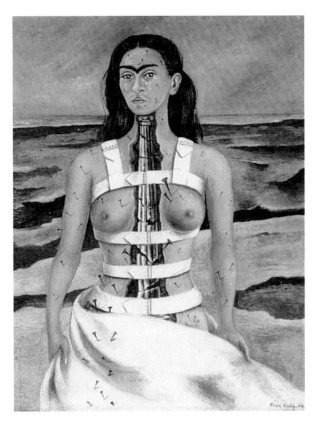

Figure 1.1 Frida Kahlo: The Broken Column (1916). Kahlo painted numerous self-portraits expressing the chronic pain she suffered subsequent to a bus accident. Reproduced with permission from Museo Dolores Olmedo Patiño, Mexico City, Mexico.

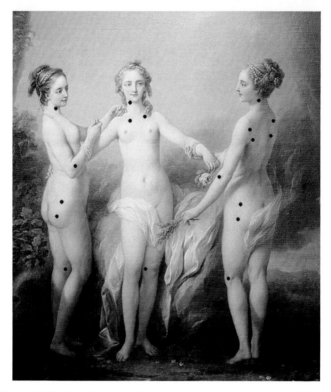

Figure 2.1 The Three Graces (Jean Baptiste van Loo) demonstrating locations of the tender points mentioned in Table 2.1. Reproduced with permission from Chateau de Chenonceau, Chenonceaux, France.

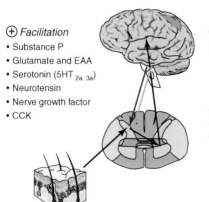

⊕ *Facilitation*
- Substance P
- Glutamate and EAA
- Serotonin (5HT$_{2a, 3a}$)
- Neurotensin
- Nerve growth factor
- CCK

⊖ *Inhibition*
- Descending antinociceptive pathways
  - Norepinephrine – serotonin (5HT$_{1a,b}$)
  - Opioids
- GABA
- Cannabanoids
- Adenosine

Figure 14.1 Influences on nociceptive processing.

Neurologic disorders

The authors have had patients with early myasthenia gravis and multiple sclerosis who were originally told they had fibromyalgia; this misdiagnosis delayed their correct diagnosis and treatment. Appropriate antibody, imaging, and electrical testing can easily make the diagnosis.

Malignancies

Early malignancies and paraneoplastic involvement can rarely present with constitutional complaints similar to those of fibromyalgia. Corticosteroids and some cancer chemotherapies (e.g., interleukin-2, interferons) also produce malaise, fatigue, and aching.

Substance abuse and malnutrition

Fatigue and pain are common in the U.S. population. Many people try to alleviate these complaints by altering their diet, increasing consumption of caffeine, or using analgesics or diet pills. Having unsound dietary regimens or consuming excessive caffeine can lead to palpitations, vitamin deficiency, and constitutional complaints of fatigue and aching. Some young women with anorexia or bulimia believe their problem is fibromyalgia and avoid confronting their psychological problem by failing to disclose this to their treating physician. Alcohol abuse and heroin use are common causes of fatigue and anxiety. Narcotic analgesics promote addiction and fatigue in the pursuit of amelioration of pain. Many patients don't tell their doctors they have a substance abuse problem when requesting help in treating what they believe to be fibromyalgia. Sudden withdrawal from alcohol, cocaine, heroin, or analgesic medications can also aggravate musculoskeletal discomfort.[2]

References

1. White KP. The differential diagnosis of chronic regional pain. In Wallace DJ, Clauw DJ, eds. *Fibromyalgia and Other Central Pain Syndromes*. Philadelphia: Lippincott Williams & Wilkins; 2005:299–308.

2. Arnold LM. Management of fibromyalgia and comorbid psychiatric disorders. *J Clin Psychiatry*. 2008;69(52):14.

Chapter 9

Methods of clinical assessment and ascertainment

Fibromyalgia patients seen in a clinical practice setting have multiple symptoms, signs, laboratory findings, and comorbidities. There is no single measure, metric, or index that allows a treating practitioner to assess, in a reliable, efficient manner, how a fibromyalgia patient is responding to a therapeutic intervention. Response to a prescribed intervention is usually assessed after listening to the patient and examining him or her. This is not sufficient in a clinical trial setting. The U.S. Food and Drug Administration has produced an industry guidance document for fibromyalgia clinical trials, and agents being studied are assessed using primary and secondary outcome measures. Pregabalin, for example, met endpoints such as a Mean Pain Score, Patient Global Impression of Change, and Fibromyalgia Impact Questionnaire. The purpose of this brief chapter is to provide the reader with a menu of methods of clinical assessment and ascertainment that have been validated to varying degrees. These methods can be used in fibromyalgia clinical trials.[1] A critical review of the specific features of these inventories is beyond the scope of this monograph, but they are summarized in Table 9.1.

Table 9.1 Inventories and methodologies used in fibromyalgia and clinical trials
1. Evaluating pain
a. Visual analogue scale
b. McGill Pain Questionnaire
c. Tender point evaluations
d. Leeds Assessment of Neuropathic Symptoms and Signs
e. Brief Pain Inventory
f. Dolorimetry
2. Patient and global impression of change
3. Fatigue
a. Multidimensional Assessment of Fatigue
b. Functional Assessment of Chronic Illness Therapy
c. Fatigue severity scale

Table 9.1 (*Continued*)

4. Sleep
    a. Medical Outcomes Sleep Scale
    b. Pittsburg Sleep Quality Index
    c. Jenkins Sleep Scale
5. Function and quality of life
    a. Fibromyalgia Impact Questionnaire
    b. Short-Form-36 (SF-36) Health Survey
    c. Health Assessment Questionnaire
    d. Sexual functioning inventories
6. Psychological evaluations
    a. Beck Depression Inventory
    b. Beck Anxiety Inventory
    c. Mini International Neuropsychiatric Interview
    d. Hospital Anxiety and Depression Scale
    e. Hamilton Depression Rating Scale
    f. Stress-Trait Anxiety Inventory
    g. Coping Strategies Questionnaire
7. Neurocognitive state (dyscognition)
8. Objective biomarkers

Reference

1. Mease PJ. Assessment of patients with fibromyalgia syndrome. *J Musculoskel Pain.* 2008;16:75–80.

Chapter 10

General concepts of treatment

As with most other chronic medical illnesses, a "disease management" approach that combines patient education and pharmacological and nonpharmacological therapy likely represents the best overall treatment program. Moreover, it is often helpful or even necessary to have a real or "virtual" team of care providers that includes physician extenders (excellent for performing follow-up visits and working with patients on implementing nondrug therapies such as exercise and cognitive-behavioral approaches). This may not be practical in all settings, but it is something that can be strived for.

Figure 10.1 shows why combining pharmacological and nonpharmacological therapies is so helpful. When individuals have chronic pain, fatigue, and other symptoms for long periods of time, they often develop high levels of distress because they cannot function normally as a parent, coworker, or spouse; markedly decrease their activity levels; and become isolated, sleep poorly, and develop maladaptive illness behaviors (bad habits that unknowingly make their symptoms worse rather than better). Research has shown that every normal individual will develop increased pain or fatigue when any of these events occur. Chronic symptoms do not typically respond to drugs but instead require a "rehab" approach, where nondrug therapies must be aggressively used to restore function. Thus, the optimal regimen for fibromyalgia and other chronic pain states is to use drug or other therapies to address the initial symptoms of pain and nondrug therapies to address the functional consequences, leading to a much better overall impact on symptoms than when either one is used alone.

This chapter reviews lifestyle changes, physical measures, psychological interventions, environmental adaptations, and alternative medication approaches. Few of these remedies or ameliorations have been validated by the methods of clinical ascertainment summarized in Chapter 9. Consequently, the writers will use an "eminence-based," as opposed to "evidence-based," approach to summarize as a consensus experience what "works."[1]

The educational session

Individuals with newly diagnosed fibromyalgia benefit greatly from an educational session that helps explain the underlying nature of fibromyalgia

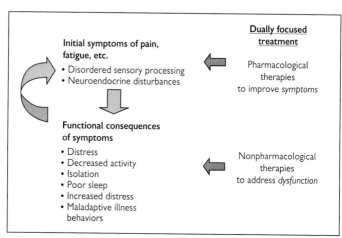

Initial symptoms of pain, fatigue, etc.

- Disordered sensory processing
- Neuroendocrine disturbances

Dually focused treatment

Pharmacological therapies
to improve *symptoms*

Functional consequences of symptoms

- Distress
- Decreased activity
- Isolation
- Poor sleep
- Increased distress
- Maladaptive illness behaviors

Nonpharmacological therapies
to address *dysfunction*

Figure 10.1 Daily focused treatment.

(e.g., it is not a problem in the areas of the body where they are experiencing pain, but rather a problem with the "volume control" setting in pain processing), as well as the value of using nonpharmacological self-management strategies along with pharmacological and other therapies. There are a number of sources of high-quality educational information on fibromyalgia from patient advocacy groups (e.g., National Fibromyalgia Association, Fibromyalgia Network, Arthritis Foundation), industry (Lilly has an excellent fibromyalgia disease management program (www.knowfibro.com)), and academic sites (e.g., the University of Michigan Chronic Pain & Fatigue Research Center Web site, www.med.umich.edu/painresearch/).

In this educational session, clinicians should explain fibromyalgia using the terms they are most comfortable with. Key concepts to reinforce are that this disorder does not cause damage to the muscles or joints, that patients must play a very active role in managing their illness, that drugs alone are rarely adequate to manage fibromyalgia, and that the overwhelming majority of patients with fibromyalgia who wish to are able to work full time. One useful analogy in this regard is to explain to patients that if they were newly diagnosed with diabetes, they would know that the treatment of diabetes does not just involve taking insulin a few times per day but rather involves exercise, diet, and an overall "disease management" approach. Every effort should be made to diminish the patient being "stigmatized" or "medicalized" as having fibromyalgia. Patients should be informed that a better prognosis is associated with improved sleep hygiene and coping strategies, stress-reduction measures, and validated exercise programs.

Lifestyle alterations

There is no specific diet for fibromyalgia, but a well-balanced, healthy one is recommended. There are no specific diets that are known to be better or worse for fibromyalgia patients. If patients feel worse when they follow a certain diet, they should avoid those foods.

Vitamin supplementation is harmless, but other than vitamin D (levels of which are low in many fibromyalgia patients, though it is not yet clear whether repletion is associated with improved symptoms), replenishment of any specific one has not been shown to be beneficial.

Smoking has been associated with lower pain thresholds in fibromyalgia patients and can aggravate dysautonomia.

Changes in barometric pressure may transiently increase stiffness and aching in vulnerable patients. No specific weather is helpful for fibromyalgia patients. Some individuals in colder climates develop a seasonal affective disorder during the winter, which can be helped by a vacation to a warmer, sunny climate.

Fatigue is a near-universal complaint of fibromyalgia patients. Lying in bed all day or working 20-hour days would be equally harmful in this regard. Patients should be introduced to the concept of "pacing," or alternating periods of activity with rest. Improving restful sleep (discussed below) and avoiding daytime naps diminish complaints of fatigue.

Fibromyalgia is a form of chronic widespread pain. There is considerable evidence that various distractions lead to not dwelling or thinking about this discomfort. This could include engaging in hobbies or pleasurable activities, listening to music, watching a movie, or any other activity that has the potential to decrease pain perception.

Improving sleep architecture without using medication

Our 640 muscles are microtraumatized daily. The healing process occurs during sleep, when melatonin and growth hormone, among other chemicals, are secreted. Failure to experience restful sleep results in more fatigue, pain, and generalized discomfort during the day. Following the rules of sleep hygiene is often more successful than using sleep aids. Improved sleep architecture is one of the most important outcome measures correlating with an improved prognosis. Some easy-to-adopt measures are listed in Table 10.1.

Optimizing the home environment

Avoiding activities that aggravate musculoskeletal pain starts with creating a safe, easy-to-use living space. Some measures that are helpful to selected fibromyalgia patients include cooking two meals at once, taking breaks between tasks, arranging activities to decrease the number of times one has to walk up and down stairs, avoiding putting items that get a lot of use in high cupboards or cabinets, raising the level of electrical plugs, and using larger handles for grasping. Rolling carts offer accessible, additional workspace and lazy Susans increase access to items. Physical and occupational

Table 10.1 Some rules of sleep hygiene

1. Sleep in a quiet room.
2. The mattress should be firm.
3. Bed partners should not snore.
4. No children or pets in the bedroom.
5. Avoid daytime napping.
6. Take a hot shower or bath in the evening before going to sleep.
7. No alcohol or caffeine after 6 p.m.
8. Avoid vigorous exercise after 6 p.m.
9. For the hour prior to retiring, avoid violent or unpleasant reading or frightening television shows or movies. Consider listening to soft, gentle music. Create a sleep-friendly home environment.
10. Go to bed at the same time every night and awaken at the same time in the morning. If unable to sleep in the middle of the night, "putter" for 30 to 45 minutes and then return to bed, awakening at the usual time.

therapists (see below) can teach patients ways to vacuum, wash dishes, or clean that minimize stress to the upper back and neck regions. The family vehicle should have a bucket seat or good lumbar support, be easy to enter and exit, and have a headrest and a good climate control system. Mirrors should be plentiful and well placed (Fig. 10.2).

Exercise and rehabilitation

Exercise and activity are essential components of fibromyalgia management. Although early studies suggested that aerobic exercise was the only type of exercise to be of benefit, more recent studies have suggested that strength training, stretching, yoga, and many other types of exercise can also be helpful.[2,3] For some patients who are very sedentary, the term "exercise" is frightening and not practical, and it is best to focus on getting these individuals to increase their daily activities (e.g., get out of bed, move, take stairs, walk short distances) before even contemplating a formal "exercise" routine.

The fundamental principles of good body mechanics in fibromyalgia involve using a broad base of support by distributing loads to stronger joints with a greater surface area, keeping items close to the body to provide leverage, not staying in the same position for a prolonged period of time, and avoiding too much pressure to tender regions. Surveys suggest that up to 80% of patients with fibromyalgia do not exercise regularly and are not physically fit. Many patients complain that fatigue and pain are worse after exertion. Deconditioning leads to osteopenia, muscle atrophy, and increased fatigue. Some studies have suggested that muscles in fibromyalgia patients are more prone to autonomically mediated vasoconstriction, which leads to localized hypoxia and discomfort with exercise (at least at first).

The best exercise program is one that emphasizes generalized conditioning and that can be performed daily or nearly every day. This includes

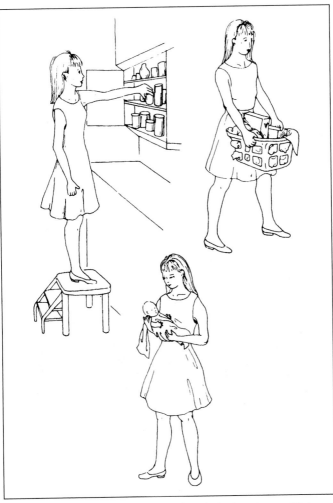

Figure 10.2 The basic principles of proper body mechanics that enhance well-being in fibromyalgia. Reprinted with permission from Wallace DJ. *Fibromyalgia: An Essential Guide for Patients and Their Families.* New York: Oxford University Press.

walking, swimming, bicycling, and low-impact aerobics, while avoiding activities that put too much pressure on the upper back and neck, such as tennis, bowling, weightlifting, rowing, or golf. Isometric (as opposed to isotonic), Pilates-based approaches and stretching exercises should be the optimal therapeutic focus for fibromyalgia patients (Fig. 10.3).

Some patients may benefit from a formal rehabilitation program, best provided by physical and occupational therapists who have had experience

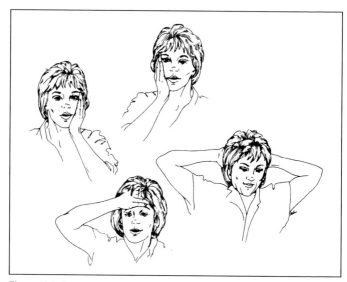

Figure 10.3 An example of strength-building isometric exercises. Reprinted with permission from Wallace DJ. *Fibromyalgia: An Essential Guide for Patients and Their Families.* New York: Oxford University Press.

working with fibromyalgia patients (therapists who typically see sports medicine patients often try to do too much too soon with fibromyalgia patients). It is important for the therapist to set up a program that the patients can then perform on their own—it is best not to have the therapist supervise all exercise, because it is not practical for patients to exercise under supervision the rest of their life.

These allied health professionals are adept at instructing patients in multiple modalities. Some of these include gentle massage, spray and stretch, moist heat (for chronic pain; ice is useful for acute strains for the first 36 hours), electrical stimulation, manipulation (also provided by chiropractors and osteopaths), posture and gait training, instruction in footwear choices, and relaxation techniques. Occupational therapists are skilled in performing an activities of daily living (ADL) evaluation that examines how patients function in their house or workplace and maneuver (e.g., getting in and out of a car or bathtub, getting on or off a toilet seat, washing dishes). By applying the principles of energy conservation and joint protection, the rehabilitation therapists may recommend the use of assistive devices (e.g., splints, braces) or workstation enhancements (e.g., computer screens at the proper height, special chairs).

Acupuncture

According to ancient Chinese tradition, *qi* (pronounced *chee*) is an energizing life force that flows in the body through meridians, or imaginary lines. Acupuncture involves inserting fine-gauge, sterilized needles along these meridians to allow "energy paths" signaling the brain to dampen pain. Results of controlled studies using acupuncture to treat fibromyalgia have been contradictory but suggest that this modality probably has a modest benefit.[4]

Behavioral modalities

Mental health specialists, allied health professionals, clergy, and complementary practitioners can alleviate many manifestations of fibromyalgia with their expertise. These professionals use a variety of techniques to decrease stress, enhance coping skills, diminish fatigue, build self-esteem, and improve interpersonal interactions.[5,6]

There are two general categories of referrals. Many patients with fibromyalgia will benefit from cognitive-behavioral therapy. This type of therapy is often provided by psychologists or social workers with specific training and can be offered in group or individual sessions. A smaller percentage of fibromyalgia patients need referral to psychiatrists or psychologists who perform psychotherapy or help manage comorbid psychiatric or psychological conditions. This would include patients with profound anxiety, depression, post-traumatic stress disorder, psychosis (e.g., bipolar illness), or complicated medication or medical issues.

The goals of psychological intervention are to promote the development of positive goals and attitudes, introduce adaptive measures to improve coping, deal with stress (e.g., deep-breathing exercises, relaxation techniques, promoting hobbies), and nurturing a positive doctor–patient relationship. Family support systems are optimized, and concerned friends and relatives are educated about fibromyalgia and how to maximize the home environment. A good sexual relationship is a source of pleasure, self-esteem, relaxation, and stress reduction.

The mind–body connection plays a major role in the management of fibromyalgia patients with cognitive dysfunction, or "fibro-fog." Interventions such as cognitive-behavioral therapy, biofeedback, electroencephalographic biofeedback, and guided imagery are usually supervised by psychologists or other allied health professionals. They manipulate sympathetically mediated vasomotor instability and introduce relaxation techniques to improve clarity of thought and decrease anxiety. Meditation, yoga, t'ai chi, and prayer are used by complementary practitioners and clergy as well.

References

1. Burckhardt CS. Nonpharmacological management strategies in fibromyalgia. *Rheum Dis North Am.* 2002;28:291–304.

2. Jones KD, Adams D, Winters-Stone K, et al. A comprehensive review of 46 exercise treatment studies in fibromyalgia (1988–2005). *Health & Quality of Life Outcome.* 2006:4:67.

3. Sim J, Adams N. Systemic review of randomized controlled trials of nonpharmacological interventions for fibromyalgia. *Clin J Pain.* 2002;18:324–336.

4. Martin DP, Sletten CD, Williams BA, et al. Improvement in fibromyalgia symptoms with acupuncture: results of a randomized controlled trial. *Mayo Clin Proc.* 2006;81:749–757.

5. Wallace DJ, Clauw DJ, Hallegua DS. Addressing behavioral abnormalities in fibromyalgia. *J Musculoskel Med.* 2005;22:562–579.

6. Koulil SV, Effting M, Kraaimaat FW, et al. Cognitive-behavioral therapies and exercise programmes for patients with fibromyalgia: state of the art and future directions. *Ann Rheum Dis.* 2007;66:571–581.

Chapter 11

Medications used to manage fibromyalgia

Treatment

Progress in the understanding of fibromyalgia has led to considerably more therapeutic options for patients with this condition.

Diagnostic labeling

Once a physician rules out other potential disorders, an important and at times controversial step in the management of fibromyalgia is asserting the diagnosis. Despite some assumptions that being "labeled" with fibromyalgia may adversely affect patients, a study by White et al. indicated that patients had significant improvement in health satisfaction and symptoms after being "labeled." Nonetheless, in select individuals (i.e., adolescents or young adults) or overtly anxious persons, the preferred route may still be not to label. Regardless, as noted above, diagnosis confirmation should be ideally coupled with patient education, an intervention shown to be effective in randomized controlled trials.

Local therapies

Most patients with myofascial pain syndrome can avoid long-term systemic therapies. Local approaches include injections and topical agents (Table 11.1). Their effectiveness has not been well studied in randomized clinical trials and may be dependent upon regional variation in drug penetration, concentration gradients, dosing schedules, and vehicles (e.g., cream, ointment, lotion, occlusive dressing).[1] All of the approaches mentioned in this section have been demonstrated to ameliorate localized pain in controlled studies. No toxicity has been reported when these are used adjunctively with agents approved by the U.S. Food and Drug Administration (FDA) for fibromyalgia.

Tender point injections

We tend to consider using local injections only when a significant component of a patient's discomfort at any given visit emanates from a single location or region. The agent of choice is an anesthetic (usually lidocaine) with or without a low dose of a corticosteroid such as methylprednisolone, betamethasone, dexamethasone, or triamcinolone. Up to 10 mL of lidocaine given in as many as four or five injections can be used at a

Table 11.1 Topical therapies used by fibromyalgia patients

- Trigger point injections
  - Lidocaine or similar agents
  - Dry needling
  - Steroids
  - Botulinum toxin
- Topical remedies
  - Salicylates
  - Nonsteroidals
  - Anticonvulsants (e.g., gabapentin)
  - Anesthetics (e.g., lidocaine)
  - Capsaicin
  - Antidepressants
  - Traditional Chinese medicines
- Physical measures
  - Massage
  - Balneotherapy
  - Heat therapy
  - Ultrasound
  - Phonopheresis
  - Local electrical stimulation (e.g., TENS)

single session. Risks include pneumothorax (if the tender region is in the upper back area) and lipoatrophy with triamcinolone. Most patients report transient relief; these injections can be given frequently if necessary. Some practitioners use dry needling as well. Occasionally, botulinum toxin is injected into tender points, with up to 3 months of relief. Used medically for strabismus and blepharospasm, controlled studies have documented benefits for Botox in the management of headache and neck pain.

Nerve blocks

Nerve blocks such as epidurals and facet blocks are frequently administered to patients with discogenic disease and spinal stenosis. These treatments are not generally recommended for fibromyalgia patients without these comorbid conditions.

Topical therapies

Compounded gels or patches containing ketoprofen, diclofenac, gabapentin, amitriptyline, and/or cyclobenzaprine have been used to treat localized pain or neuritic symptoms. Mild discomfort is relieved with aspirin-containing over-the-counter preparations with or without the soothing effects of camphor or menthol. Capsaicin, a cayenne pepper derivative that depletes substance P, is approved by the FDA for osteoarthritis pain but seems to help only a small number of fibromyalgia patients. Topical anesthetics in preparations such as lidocaine patches may be quite successful in treating localized pain.

Additional topical and physical measures and devices

Some practitioners use topical traditional Chinese medicine. Physical therapists employ heat, ultrasound, phonopheresis (using ultrasound to drive pharmacologic agents such as corticosteroids or lidocaine subdermally into subcutaneous tissues), and transcutaneous electrical nerve stimulation (TENS). Balneotherapy, which involves bathing in mineral-containing waters or hot springs or the use of mud baths, has been shown to be effective in randomized controlled trials. Although most of these interventions have not been studied using adequate evidence-based methodologies, they are generally harmless, and some patients report considerable benefits.

Medications used to treat fibromyalgia

In 2005, the FDA summarized the results of hearings and issued a guidance document to industry that established a roadmap for drugs to receive approval for a fibromyalgia indication. As of June 2009, three agents have been approved by the FDA for fibromyalgia. Before 2005, hundreds of fibromyalgia clinical trials were conducted using widely varying methodologies, rigor, and design. This following section reviews how these agents are viewed and used.

Agents where efficacy has been validated in large-scale, double-blind, placebo-controlled trials

Pregabalin (Lyrica) is a ligand for alpha-2-delta subtype 1 and 2 receptors that adheres to voltage-gated calcium channels and reduces calcium flux in neurons.[2] This reduces the release of substance P, glutamate, and norepinephrine, resulting in analgesia and less anxiety. Using the Mean Pain Score as the primary endpoint and Patient Global Impression of Change and the Fibromyalgia Impact Questionnaire as secondary endpoints, just about half of patients had a 30% response in doses of 300 to 600 mg daily.[3] Major side effects included dizziness, somnolence, weight gain, and edema. Many practitioners have found that some patients do well with doses as low as 75 mg daily. Gabapentin is a similar compound that has also been shown in a single large controlled study to be effective in fibromyalgia; doses of 1600 to 2400 mg are often necessary to show an analgesic effect. Patients often tolerate these compounds much better if most or all of the drug is given at bedtime (Fig. 11.1).

Duloxetine (Cymbalta) is a serotonin/norepinephrine reuptake inhibitor (SNRI) that has been on the market in the United States for generalized anxiety disorder, diabetic neuropathy, and depression since 2005. In approximately 1,500 patients enrolled in four pivotal fibromyalgia trials, pain, global impression, fatigue, and function were shown to improve. The studies showed that both 60 and 120 mg were effective doses (Fig. 11.2). All SNRIs and norepinephrine/serotonin reuptake inhibitors (NSRIs) have a similar side effect profile, with nausea, constipation, postural dizziness, and palpitations as common adverse reactions. The nausea may be reduced by taking the drug with food, and the other side effects are often self-limited

- Pooled analysis of two 14-week monotherapy trials

  - N = PBO (374), 300 mg (368), 450 (373), or 600 (378) mg/d
  - Primary endpoint: mean pain score (MPS)
  - Patient global impression of change (PGIC) and Fibromyalgia Impact Questionnaire (FIQ) key secondary measures

- Pain and PGIC stat sig at all three doses, FIQ at 450 and 600

- AEs: dizziness, somnolence, and weight gain

- Key points

  - Further supportive data regarding efficacy and tolerability from large data set used for FDA approval of pregabalin for the management of FM
  - These pain responder rates are typical for trials of pain medications in a variety of pain conditions

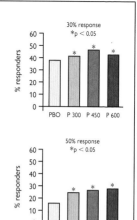

Figure 11.1 FM treatment: pregabalin. Adapted from Duan R, et al. *71st ACR*, Boston 2007. Abstract #1524.

Study	Dose (mg/d)	Wks	Dul (N)	PBO (N)	Efficacy outcomes at 3 months			
					BPI average pain	BPI 30% improvement	BPI 50% improvement	PGI improvement
Study 1 Phase II	120	12	101	103	+	NS	+	+
Study 2 Phase III Women	60 120	12	118 116	120	+ +	+ +	+ +	+ +
Study 3 Phase III	20 60 120	28	79 150 147	144	NS + +	NS + +	NS NS +	NS + +
Study 4 Phase III	60/120	27	162	168	NS	NS	NS	NS

Figure 11.2 FM treatment: duloxetine—a serotonin/norepinephrine reuptake inhibitor (SNRI). Adapted from Chappell A, et al. *71st ACR*, Boston 2007. Abstract #1543; Arnold LM, et al. *Pain*. 2005;119:5–15; Russell IJ, et al. *Musculoskel Pain*. 2007; 15(Suppl 13):58.

and dissipate with time; they can be minimized by starting at a low dose and escalating slowly.

Milnacipran (Savella), a norepinephrine/serotonin reuptake inhibitor (NSRI) that has been used to manage depression for some time in Europe and Japan, was approved by the FDA for use in fibromyalgia in adults in early 2009. Milnacipran's efficacy was established in two large double-blind, placebo-controlled multicenter studies. Significant improvements were found in pain, patient global assessment, and physical function. This compound showed similar overall effects to duloxetine, with additional possible benefits in treating the cognitive problems often seen in fibromyalgia. These effects occurred at both 100 and 200 mg per day; patients are usually begun on 12.5 mg a day and the dose is titrated to therapeutic levels over a 1- to 2-week period (Fig. 11.3).

Tricyclic antidepressants

Tricyclic antidepressants (TCAs) may ameliorate the symptoms of fibromyalgia through their reuptake inhibition of serotonin and norepinephrine, but additional possible mechanisms of action include improvement of the alpha-delta wave sleep abnormality, or effects mediated via *N*-methyl d-aspartate antagonism and/or sodium channel blocking activity. In our experience, approximately one third of patients given a TCA report improvement in their fibromyalgia symptoms. Principal side effects of TCAs include sicca symptoms, fatigue, and weight gain. TCAs tend to be effective as analgesics at much lower doses than those used to manage clinical depression. In 2005, Arnold critically reviewed 21 double-blind, placebo-controlled TCA trials published since 1986 with amitriptyline, cyclobenzaprine, nortriptyline, and trazodone.[4] The most commonly used outcome measures

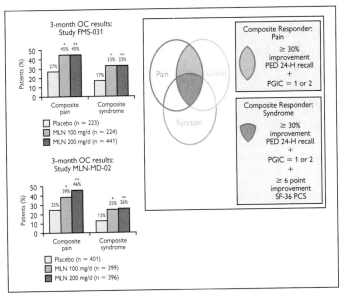

Figure 11.3 Milnacipran—a noradrenaline/serotonin reuptake inhibitor (NSRI). Adapted from Clauw D, et al. *71st ACR*, Boston 2007. Abstract #716; Clauw D et al. *71st ACR*, Boston 2007. Abstract #L1; Goldenberg at al. *71st ACR*, Boston 2007. Abstract #1526.

included pain, visual analogue scales, physician global assessments, fatigue scales, dolorimetry, pain inventories, tender point examinations, tenderness measurements, and quality-of-life questionnaires. Four of the studies had a negative outcome; 17 demonstrated statistically significant responses using at least two of the metrics.

Selective serotonin reuptake inhibitors

Selective serotonin reuptake inhibitors (SSRIs) primarily increase levels of serotonin, but some of these compounds (e.g.m fluoxetine, paroxetine, sertraline) also increase norepinephrine, especially at higher doses. In contrast, the newer SSRIs, such as citalopram and escitalopram, are highly selective reuptake inhibitors that do not appreciably increase norepinephrine levels; because of this, they are less effective as analgesics. Studies of the use of these commonly prescribed agents as monotherapy for fibromyalgia have generally been disappointing.

Dopaminergic agents

Pramipexole and ropinirole are D3 receptor agonists approved for use in restless legs syndrome. Several controlled trials have suggested improved scores on assessments of pain, fatigue, function, and global status, especially in narcotic-dependent or disabled patients in fibromyalgia. Anxiety, compulsive behavior, and weight loss may occur. This may be a useful class of drugs in patients with comorbid restless legs syndrome.

Muscle relaxants

Carisoprodol, orphenadrine, and metaxalone have been prescribed for over 30 years as non-drowsiness-inducing muscle relaxants with subjective benefit, but they have never been seriously studied in fibromyalgia.

Benzodiazepines

Benzodiazepines diminish the alpha-delta wave sleep abnormality, improve sleep myoclonus, are anxiolytic, and inhibit the transmission of excitatory nerve impulses by increasing levels of gamma-aminobutyric acid (GABA). Only one randomized controlled trial has been performed using a benzodiazepine, and it was found to be ineffective. Anecdotally, many clinicians avoid this class of drugs in fibromyalgia because other compounds are more efficacious and do not disrupt sleep architecture. Nevertheless, many practitioners use alprazolam to manage daytime anxiety, lorazepam to treat anxiety-related insomnia, clonazepam to promote sleep and muscle relaxation, or diazepam for muscle spasm and anxiety. There are no evidence-based studies supporting their use.

Anticonvulsants

Lamotrigine, topiramate, carbamazepine, levetiracetam, and mexiletine have been used off label for numbness, burning, tingling, depression, anxiety, and headaches associated with fibromyalgia via sodium or calcium channel blockade and increasing GABA levels. There are no evidence-based studies supporting their use.

Sedative–hypnotic medications

Although zolpidem, eszopiclone, and temazepam are approved for insomnia and zolpidem improves sleep architecture abnormalities associated with fibromyalgia, they have no documented effect on pain. In contrast, sodium oxybate is a potent precursor of GABA available for restricted use for narcolepsy, and it has been shown to improve both pain and sleep in fibromyalgia. However, its efficacy is tempered by its potential for abuse, especially as a "date rape" agent.

Nonsteroidal anti-inflammatory agents (NSAIDs), salicylates, and acetaminophen

In patients without a comorbid "peripheral" pain syndrome such as osteoarthritis, NSAIDs do not appear to be very efficacious in fibromyalgia, especially as monotherapy. Salicylates are used in many topical preparations (see above). Acetaminophen has not been studied, but its usefulness is limited at best.

Opiates

A survey of academic medical centers found that 14% of fibromyalgia patients were taking opiates, even though there are no controlled trials showing that opioids are effective in fibromyalgia. An increasing problem in clinical practice is that fibromyalgia patients are placed on opioids and stay on them for long periods, despite a lack of documentation of improvement in pain or function. Although it can often be very difficult to get these patients off opioids, one approach that can be helpful is to ask the patients if they really feel these drugs are improving their pain; when they respond negatively, as they typically do, the clinician can suggest that these drugs be slowly tapered and replaced with more efficacious classes of drugs.

Tramadol

Tramadol is a novel analgesic with weak agonist activity via the mu opioid receptor and dual serotonin and norepinephrine reuptake inhibition. It has been shown in two randomized controlled trials to be slightly effective in fibromyalgia, both alone and in combination with acetaminophen.

Management of fatigue using stimulants

Few agents have been shown specifically to reduce fatigue in fibromyalgia. As noted above, the dual reuptake inhibitors such as milnacipran and duloxetine may be helpful in treating this symptom. Weak stimulants such as modafinil or bupropion may also be helpful, although there are no good data supporting this in fibromyalgia patients. In our anecdotal experience, more powerful stimulants such as amphetamines have generally not been useful.

Other agents

NMDA antagonists such as *dextromethorphan* might have minimal effects, and *ketamine* is too toxic for routine use in fibromyalgia. In general, the use of NMDA antagonists has been disappointing in pain patients because it appears as though adequately blocking the actions of this receptor leads to

Table 11.2 Associated fibromyalgia central sensitization syndromes that may require additional treatments
1. Irritable bowel and non-ulcer dyspepsia
2. Dysautonomia
3. Dysmenorrhea
4. Irritable bladder/interstitial cystitis
5. Tension headache

too many untoward side effects. Many drugs are in development, however, that act similarly by blocking the activity of glutamate in the central nervous system.

Tizanidine (*Zanaflex*) activates alpha-2 adrenergic receptors that control sympathetic nervous system discharges, and some studies have suggested that is has mild efficacy in fibromyalgia, although there are better data that it has muscle relaxant effects.

Adjunctive agents

Most fibromyalgia patients have at least one other central sensitivity syndrome, such as irritable bowel syndrome, tension headache, interstitial cystitis, and a number of other conditions. Remedies for specific complaints related to these associated syndromes are frequently used concomitantly with fibromyalgia medications (Table 11.2). A discussion of these approaches is beyond the scope of this monograph.

Complementary and alternative medicine (CAM)

Nearly $27 billion is spent annually in the United States on CAM, 40% of which represents an out-of-pocket expense. Over 90% of fibromyalgia patients have used topical agents, massage, chiropractic therapy, homeopathy, or acupuncture or gone on special diets at one time or another, and 40% try at least one approach in any given year. Despite this, very few randomized clinical trials have examined the efficacy of any of these interventions.[5]

CAM treatments and modalities are divided into categories that are enumerated in Table 11.3. Those that work with the mind–body connection, such as meditation, guided imagery, yoga, or other relaxation techniques, modulate the autonomic nervous system and tend to be effective in some fibromyalgia patients. Approaches involving physical efforts (e.g., Pilates, chiropractic) can be useful if proper attention is given to the body mechanics reviewed in Chapter 10. Finally, herbs, vitamins, supplements, and special diets have not been subjected to the rigor necessary to demonstrate their usefulness. Sometimes, a sympathetic practitioner who is reassuring can end up helping the patient as much as the supplements he or

Table 11.3 Examples of complementary and alternative medicine used for fibromyalgia that have been evaluated in peer-reviewed literature

- Mantipulative, physical, and manual modalities
  - Acupuncture*
  - Alexander technique
  - Chiropractic
  - Feldenkrais therapy*
  - Massage*
  - Osteopathy
  - Reflexology
  - T'ai chi
  - Yoga
- Detoxification regimens
  - Chelation therapy
  - Colonic irrigation
  - Magnet therapy
- Mental modalities
  - Aromatherapy
  - Autogenic training*
  - Biofeedback*
  - Cognitive-behavioral therapy*
  - Guided imagery*
  - Hypnotherapy*
  - Meditation
  - Prayer
  - Spiritual healing
- Herbal, dietary, and "nutraceutical" approaches
  - Magnesium supplements at 500 to 1000 mg per day
  - Folk remedies
  - Naturopathy
  - Ascorbigen
  - Co-enzyme Q10
  - Gingko biloba
  - Chlorella pyrenoidosa
  - S-adenosyl methionine*
  - Vitamins B_6, B_{12}, C, D
  - Echinacea
  - Evening primrose
  - l-tryptophan
  - Peppermint
  - St. John's wort*
  - Valerian root
  - Melatonin*

*Controlled studies suggest some benefit.

she recommends. Musculoskeletal specialists tend to take a "do no harm" approach when asked about supplements by patients. Since they are not subject to scrutiny by regulatory agencies, these preparations may or may not have the amount of product listed on their label and could have sensitizing preservatives, which also interfere with absorption.

Summary

A multidisciplinary approach to managing fibromyalgia is shown in Table 11.4. Most fibromyalgia patients who have not gone on disability and are not taking high doses of narcotics will have documented improvements in their symptoms and signs when managed by a knowledgeable, caring practitioner.

Table 11.4 Treatment approach for fibromyalgia

1. Does the patient fulfill criteria for fibromyalgia? If yes, then:
   a. Consider whether label may be harmful (e.g., in adolescents or in patients with high levels of anxiety about the diagnosis).
   b. Educate the patient about the syndrome.
   c. Establish the presence of and address any medical or psychiatric comorbidities.
2. Review non-medication treatment modalities such as:
   a. Sleep hygiene instruction
   b. Principles of exercise
   c. Cognitive-behavioral therapies such as pacing, relaxation, pleasant activity scheduling, etc.
3. Is the syndrome prominent in a single region of the body?
   a. Assess the usefulness of more local therapies such as injection, topical applications, or physical or occupational therapy.
4. Is fibromyalgia affecting the patient's quality of life to the point that medication is indicated? If so, consider the following therapies:
   a. SNRI/NSRI alone (duloxetine, milnacipran) for patients with comorbid depression or prominent fatigue
   b. TCAs at bedtime
   c. Pregabalin alone (perhaps for patients with prominent sleep disturbances)
   d. Any of the classes of drugs in a, b, and c can be used in combination.
   e. Consider using other classes of drugs noted above with less well-documented efficacy.
5. Address and treat associated central sensitivity syndromes such as tension headache, functional bowel syndrome, or chronic pelvic region pain.
6. Address and treat autonomic symptoms.
7. Consider consulting a musculoskeletal or pain specialist versed in managing fibromyalgia and/or referring the patient to a psychiatrist or psychologist to manage comorbid psychiatric conditions.

References

1. Meyer HP. Myofascial pain syndrome and its suggested role in the pathogenesis and treatment of fibromyalgia syndrome. *Curr Pain Headache Rep.* 2002;6: 274–283.

2. Holman AJ. Treatment of fibromyalgia: a changing of the guard. *Women's Health.* 2005;1:409–420.

3. Crofford LJ, Rowbotham MC, Mease PJ, et al.; Pregabalin 1008–105 Study Group. Pregabalin for the treatment of fibromyalgia syndrome: results of a randomized, double-blind, placebo-controlled trial. *Arthritis Rheum.* 2005;52:1264–1273.

4. Arnold LM. Systemic therapies for chronic pain. In: Wallace DJ, Clauw DJ. *Fibromyalgia and other central pain syndromes.* Philadelphia: Lippincott Williams & Wilkins, 2005:365–388.

5. Berman BM, Swyers JP. Complementary medicine treatments for fibromyalgia syndrome. *Baillieres Best Clin Prac Res Clin Rheumatol.* 1999;13:487–492.

Chapter 12

Economic impact and disability issues

While many initiatives have scrutinized the financial impact of chronic pain, other than back pain, few studies have addressed the economic burden of musculoskeletal pain or fibromyalgia per se on society. Most of the published surveys in this area concern themselves with disability.[1]

Economic burden of fibromyalgia

In the mid-1990s, a Congressional committee estimated that the direct and indirect costs of fibromyalgia in the United States were $12 billion to $14 billion a year. This contrasts with approximately 10 million office visits in the United States to physicians for pain, and $100 billion spent annually overall to treat it. It accounts for a loss of 1% to 2% of the nation's productivity. Canadian data suggested that the annual health insurance costs for fibromyalgia patients were double those of beneficiaries without fibromyalgia. A 2007 U.S. survey reported that health care costs were triple those of beneficiaries without fibromyalgia, largely due to high levels of comorbidities and health care utilization.[2]

Economic impact on productivity and disability

Half of all lost work productivity time in the United States is due to depression. In a sampling of 28,902 workers over a 2-week period, 13% lost productive work due to pain. Fibromyalgia complaints accounted for one-sixth of this (the most common cause was headache). In Finland, an employed fibromyalgia patient has a 1.4- to 1.5-fold risk of medically certified absence due to sickness not accounted for by coexisting psychiatric illness or rheumatoid arthritis. Preexisting psychosocial factors can predict the development of new-onset widespread pain after being hired for a physical job. These include low job satisfaction, low social support, and monotonous work.

Epidemiology of disability in fibromyalgia

Ninety percent of patients with fibromyalgia in the United States who wish to work are employed full time. The employment figure drops to 60% if housewives, househusbands, and retired persons are included. Among working patients with fibromyalgia, 40% have had to change their job or alter their job description to accommodate their musculoskeletal pain. In university-based, tertiary fibromyalgia referral centers, 25% of 1500 fibromyalgia patients had received disability payments at some time and 15% were on Social Security Disability. In the United States, 6% to 15% of all fibromyalgia patients are on some form of disability, in contrast with 2% of the entire non-retirement-age population. Fibromyalgia accounts for 9% of all disability payments in Canada, and 25% of Swedes with fibromyalgia are receiving disability.

Why may fibromyalgia patients be disabled?

Disability has been defined as a "limitation of function that compromises the ability to perform an activity within a range considered normal." This falls into pathology, impairment, functional, and disability domains using enablement–disablement models that include subjective factors (e.g., pain, fatigue), objective factors (e.g., synovitis, blood pressure readings), and work categories (e.g., light, medium, sedentary).[3] An individual can be temporarily or permanently totally or partially disabled. The conundrum is that disability is difficult to quantitate or measure in fibromyalgia, and none of the methodologies currently being used to assess disability apply. Part of this relates to the failure of metrics to adequately assess fatigue, stamina, subjective discomfort, and psychosocial stressors among other factors and come up with a statistically validated composite score. Currently used disability intake forms are useless in fibromyalgia patients (e.g., "Can you lift 10 pounds always, never, or occasionally?"). An examination of the 10% of fibromyalgia patients who are permanently disabled shows inability to deal with pain, poor cognitive function, severe fatigue, stress, damp work environments, low self-esteem, lower socioeconomic levels, and hopelessness.

Who is responsible for disability?

Disability must take into account predisposing factors (e.g., stressful life events, personality, chronic medical illnesses), precipitating factors (e.g., infection, trauma, emotional stress), and perpetuating factors (e.g., not liking work, untreated psychiatric illnesses). Unfortunately, these are rarely the fault of the employer, but in a worker's compensation system, all too often the employer is left holding the bag.

Preventing disability

Once fibromyalgia patients go on disability, this often leads to a downhill course of the illness.[4] One study showed a significant increase in loss of material possessions (e.g., a car); loss of support by friends and family; loss of recreational activities; decreased standard of living; disconnection with intimate partners; loss of hobbies; and reduced self-esteem, independence, and socialization. When patients go on disability there is often a concomitant decrease in physical activity and exercise that likely compounds this problem.

Fibromyalgia patients should view themselves not as disabled but as "differently abled." How can their work environment be improved to allow them to continue working? Patients should be up front with their employer and state, "This is what I can do, and do well"; they should also

Table 12.1 Disability in fibromyalgia: Summary points

1. Fibromyalgia is responsible for a 1% to 2% decrease in U.S. productivity and results in direct and indirect expenditures of at least $15 billion a year.

2. Ninety percent of fibromyalgia patients who wish to are working full time. Ten percent to 25% of working fibromyalgia patients have received disability payments at some time, and 40% have changed jobs or job descriptions due to the syndrome.

3. Ten percent of patients with fibromyalgia are permanently totally disabled, usually due to inability to deal with severe pain or fatigue or cognitive dysfunction. Most have a history of low self-esteem, anxiety, depression, and low educational attainment before employment. True work-induced disability is very rare.

4. Methods of work ability ascertainment for fibromyalgia are lacking, and current metrics are not valid for the syndrome.

5. Patient education, rehabilitation, and workstation ergonomic assistance can keep most at-risk fibromyalgia patients in the workforce, and individuals who are given total disability usually deteriorate psychologically and functionally.

pace themselves with periods of activity alternating with periods of rest and use coping strategies. Physical therapy, occupational therapy, counseling, vocational training, and ergonomic work station assessments can make a difference (Table 12.1).

References

1. Wallace DJ, Hallegua DS. Quality-of-life, legal-financial and disability issues in fibromyalgia. *Curr Pain Headache Rep.* 2001;5:313–319.

2. Berger A, Dukes E, Martin S, et al. Characteristics and healthcare costs of patients with fibromyalgia. *Int J Clin Practice.* 2007;61:1498–1508.

3. Harkness EF, Macfarlane GJ, Nahit E, et al. Mechanical injury and psychosocial factors in the workplace predict the onset of widespread body pain. *Arthritis Rheum.* 2005;50:1655–1664.

4. Wallace DJ. The economic impact of fibromyalgia on society and disability issues. In Wallace DJ, Clauw DJ, eds. *Fibromyalgia and Other Central Pain Syndromes.* Philadelphia: Lippincott Williams & Wilkins; 2005:395–400.

Chapter 13

Prognosis

Relatively few studies have examined the outcome of myofascial pain and fibromyalgia. Results vary widely depending on the clinical setting where patients were seen, who saw them, and the length of follow-up.[1]

Outcome of myofascial pain

If appropriately treated within a short time of diagnosis, myofascial pain syndrome has an excellent prognosis, with over 75% of patients having little or no discomfort when seen 2 to 3 years later. On the other hand, in a survey of 53 patients with nondiscogenic low back pain followed by musculoskeletal specialists, 25% were diagnosed with fibromyalgia over an 18-year period. This suggests that undertreated myofascial pain can become chronic widespread pain.[2]

Outcome of fibromyalgia

Fibromyalgia is not associated with increased mortality. When diagnosed and treated by a community primary care physician, up to half of fibromyalgia patients no longer fulfilled ACR criteria for the syndrome after 2 years.[3,4] On the other hand, fewer than 2% of fibromyalgia patients seen at tertiary care centers had a favorable outcome at 2 years, and pain was rated as moderate to severe by 60% of these patients. This reinforces the concept of the importance of early diagnosis and treatment. In one study, 73% of children managed by pediatric rheumatologists no longer had significant symptoms 2 years later.

Factors associated with a poorer outcome include the presence of severe mood or behavioral disturbances, substance abuse, poor insight into the sources of psychosocial stressors, failure to graduate from high school, and being over the age of 40 when diagnosed.

References

1. Macfarlane GJ, Thomas E, Papageorgiu AC, et al. The natural history of chronic pain in the community: a better prognosis than in the clinic? *J Rheumatol.* 1996;23:1617–1620.

2. L'apossy E, Maleltzke R, Hrycaj P, et al. The frequency of transition of low back pain to fibromyalgia. *Scand J Rheumatol.* 1995;24:29–33.

3. Granges G, Zilko P, Littlejohn GO. Fibromyalgia syndrome: assessment of the severity of the condition two years after diagnosis. *J Rheumatol.* 1994;21:523–529.

4. Baumgartner E, Finchk A, Cedraschi C, et al. A six-year prospective study of a cohort of patients with fibromyalgia. *Ann Rheum Dis.* 2002;61:644–645.

Chapter 14

Experimental and innovative therapies

Within the past few years there has been an explosion of interest in fibromyalgia, within both the academic community and the pharmaceutical and device industries.

Pharmacological therapies

Figure 14.1 shows that there are a number of neurotransmitters that either increase or decrease pain and sensory transmission, and there are data suggesting that many of these neurochemicals are abnormal in fibromyalgia in a direction (i.e., elevated concentrations of the neurotransmitters on the left or too little of those on the right) that would cause a heightened state of pain or sensory processing.

Thus, any drug that acts as an antagonist of neurotransmitters on the left, or an agonist of a neurotransmitter on the right, might be effective in treating at least a subset of fibromyalgia patients who develop their heightened pain sensitivity in part because of this underlying abnormality. (The only known exception to this is that it appears as though the opioidergic

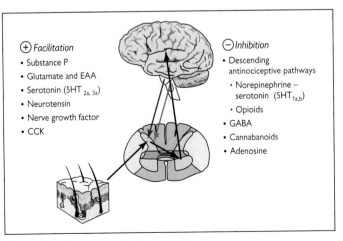

Figure 14.1 Influences on nociceptive processing.

systems are maximally activated in fibromyalgia patients, which may explain why opioidergic drugs show little efficacy in this and related conditions.) In fact, just recently a study showed that a synthetic cannabinoid was efficacious in a number of symptom domains in fibromyalgia.

Neurostimulatory therapies

Several recent studies suggest that therapies that stimulate specific brain or nervous system structures can improve pain and other symptoms in fibromyalgia. These include transcranial magnetic stimulation and direct current stimulation, two therapies that stimulate underlying brain regions using magnetic influences or direct current. These therapies appear to be well tolerated in early studies, although there is a theoretical risk of inducing seizures. Other similar therapies such as vagal nerve stimulation are also under study in fibromyalgia.

Suggested reading

1. Clauw DJ. Pharmacotherapy for patients with fibromyalgia. *J Clin Psychiatry.* 2008;69(Suppl 2):25–29.

2. Hsu MC, Clauw DJ. A different type of procedure for a different type of pain. *Arthritis Rheum.* 2006;54:3725–3727.

Resource information

The Web sites of the organizations listed below can be readily accessed through any search engine.

Nonprofit organizations

The following nonprofit organizations fund fibromyalgia research and training or promote patient advocacy and education and have a budget of over $1 million a year. Some also publish peer-reviewed journals.

Arthritis Foundation
P.O. Box 7669. Atlanta, GA 30357, 800-283-7800. There are 56 U.S. chapters that provide research monies, publish literature, and offer patient support for arthritis and related conditions such as lupus. Web site: www.arthritis.org

American College of Rheumatology (ACR)
1800 Century Place, Suite 250, Atlanta, GA 30345, 404-633-3777. This is the professional organization to which nearly all U.S. and many international rheumatologists belong. Web site: www.rheumatology.org

Research and Education Foundation of the American College of Rheumatology
1800 Century Place #250, Atlanta, GA 30345, 800-346-4753. The research-funding arm of the ACR funds rheumatology training and research programs that are vital to the care of patients with rheumatic diseases. Web site: www.rheumatology.org

National Institute of Arthritis and Musculoskeletal and Skin Diseases (NIAMS)
Bldg. 31, Room 4C05, 31 Center Drive MSC 2350, Bethesda, MD 20892, 301-496-8190. Part of the National Institutes of Health, NIAMS funds $2 million to $3 million in fibromyalgia research each year at the Bethesda campus and elsewhere in the country. Web site: www.niams.nih.gov

Fibromyalgia Network
P.O. Box 31750, Tucson, AZ 85751–1750, 520–290-5508 or 800-853-2929. Supports research through the American Fibromyalgia Syndrome Association. Web site: www.fmnetnews.com/

American Pain Society
4700 W. Lake Ave., Glenview, IL 6002, 847-375-4715, fax 877-734-8758. Multidisciplinary organization of professional pain specialists. It publishes the *Journal of Pain*. Web site: www.ampainsoc.org

National Fibromyalgia Association
2121 S. Towne Centre Place, Suite 300, Anaheim, CA 92806, 714-921-0150, fax 714–921-6920. The largest membership organization for fibromyalgia patients in the United States. Web site: www.fmaware.org

Rheumatology textbooks

Hochberg MC, Silman AJ, Smolen JS, et al., eds. *Rheumatology* (2-volume set, 4th ed.). Elsevier; 2007.

Firrestein GS, Budd RC, Hanes ED, et al., eds. *Kelley's Textbook of Rheumatology.* WB Saunders; 2008.

Isenberg D, Maddison PJ, Woo P, et al., eds. *Oxford Textbook of Rheumatology* (3d ed.). Oxford University Press; 2004.

Koopman WJ, Moreland LW. *Arthritis and Allied Conditions: A Textbook of Rheumatology* (15th ed.). Philadelphia: Lippincott Williams & Wilkins; 2004.

Wallace DJ, Clauw DJ, eds. *Fibromyalgia and other Central Pain Syndromes.* Philadelphia: Lippincott Williams & Wilkins; 2005.

Medical journals

Annals of the Rheumatic Diseases
Journal of Musculoskeletal Pain
Journal of Rheumatology
Rheumatology

Books for fibromyalgia patients

Fransen J, Russell IJ. *The Fibromyalgia Help Book: Practical Guide to Living Better with Fibromyalgia.* Smith House; 1996.

Matallana L, Bradley LA, Silverman S, Yunus M. *The Complete Idiot's Guide to Fibromyalgia.* Alpha; 2005.

Staud R, Adamec D. *Fibromyalgia for Dummies.* Wiley; 2007.

Wallace DJ, Wallace JB. *Fibromyalgia: An Essential Guide for Patients and Their Families.* New York, London: Oxford University Press; 2003.

Appendix 2

Glossary

acetylcholine: neurotransmitter of the autonomic nervous system (see below) that induces dilation of blood vessels and slows down the gastrointestinal and urinary tracts

affective spectrum disorder: term used to consider irritable bowel, tension headache, irritable bladder, premenstrual tension, and fibromyalgia as being primarily of behavioral and secondarily of physiologic causation

afferent nerves: nerves going from the periphery (e.g., skin, muscle) toward the spine

alexithymia: longstanding personality disorder with generalized and localized complaints in individuals who cannot express underlying psychological conflicts

allodynia: condition whereby something that should not hurt causes pain; fibromyalgia is chronic, widespread allodynia

alpha–delta sleep wave abnormality: delta waves make up most of slow wave, or nondream, sleep. Alpha waves interrupting delta waves can produce movement or awakening, leading to unrefreshing sleep.

American College of Rheumatology (ACR): professional association of 5000 American rheumatologists and 2000 allied health professionals (the Association of Rheumatology Health Professionals)

Arthritis Foundation: nonprofit national organization that provides patient support and funds research on musculoskeletal disorders

autonomic nervous system (ANS): part of the peripheral nervous system; divided into sympathetic and parasympathetic components. Regulates stress responses, sweat, urine, and bowel reflexes and determines whether a blood vessel constricts or dilates, thereby affecting pulse and blood pressure.

B cell: white blood cell that makes antibodies

benzodiazepines: anxiolytic group of drugs, including diazepam (Valium) and clonazepam (Klonopin), that relax muscles, among other actions, by blocking GABA (see below)

biofeedback: training technique enabling an individual to gain some voluntary control over autonomic body functions

body dysmorphic disorder: condition in which an individual is engrossed with himself or herself and/or expresses excessive concern or fear over having a defect in appearance

bradykinins: chemicals that mediate inflammation and dilate blood vessels

bruxism: persistently grinding one's teeth

bursa: sac of synovial fluid between tendons, muscles, and bones that promotes easier movement

Candida hypersensitivity syndrome: controversial condition based on theories that a toxin released by yeast is responsible for irritable bowel, fatigue, and a feeling of illness. *Candida* is a type of yeast.

carpal tunnel syndrome: compression of the median nerve as it traverses the palmar side of the wrist, producing shooting nerve pains in the first to fourth fingers

cartilage: connective tissue, often adjacent to or covering bone

causalgia: sustained burning pain, allodynia, and overreaction to stimuli associated with autonomic nervous system dysfunction. Reflex sympathetic dystrophy is chronic, widespread causalgia.

Centers for Disease Control and Prevention (CDC): an agency of the federal government based in Atlanta, Georgia, that monitors, defines, and sets standards for managing epidemics, infections, new diseases, and certain types of blood tests

central sensitization syndrome: group of local and systemic syndromes characterized by amplification of sensory afferent input resulting in pain

chiropractic: therapy involving manipulation of spine and joints to influence the body's nervous system and natural defense mechanisms

chronic fatigue immune dysfunction syndrome (CFIDS): controversial term for chronic fatigue syndrome implying a prominent role for immune abnormalities

chronic fatigue syndrome (CFS): unexplained fatigue lasting more than 6 months associated with musculoskeletal and systemic symptoms. Most CFS patients fulfill the criteria for fibromyalgia.

cognitive-behavioral therapy: use of biofeedback-related techniques to improve speech and memory

cognitive dysfunction: difficulty focusing, remembering names or dates, performing numerical calculations, or articulating clearly

collagen: structural protein found in bone, cartilage, and skin

conversion reaction: form of hysteria whereby an emotion is transformed into a physical manifestation (e.g., a person with normal vision claiming, "I can't see")

corticosteroid: any anti-inflammatory hormone made by the adrenal gland's cortex

corticotropin-releasing hormone (CRH): a chemical made in the hypothalamus of the brain that ultimately leads to the release of steroids by the adrenal gland

cortisone: a synthetic corticosteroid

costochondritis: irritation of the tethering tissues connecting the sternum (breastbone) to the ribs, producing chest pains; also called Tietze syndrome

cytokines: proteins that act as messenger chemicals of the immune system

delta sleep: a type of electrical wave found on a tracing of brain waves during non-dream sleep

depression: helplessness and hopelessness leading to feelings of worthlessness, loss of appetite, alterations in sleep patterns, loss of self-esteem, inability to concentrate, fatigue, and/or loss of energy

disability: a limitation of function that compromises one's ability to perform an activity within a range considered normal

dorsal horn: nerves inside the back of the spinal cord; runs from the brain to the waist area

dorsal root ganglion: nerve cell bodies in the peripheral nervous system that receive nociceptive inputs and transmit them to the spinal cord

dynorphin: an opiate that suppresses acute pain but perpetuates chronic pain

dysautonomia abnormal function of the autonomic nervous system

dysmenorrhea: painful periods

edema: swelling of tissues, usually due to inflammation or fluid retention

efferent nerves: nerves that go from the spinal cord to its periphery

electroencephalogram (EEG): map of electrical activity within the brain

electromyogram (EMG): map of electrical activity within muscles; usually combined with a *nerve conduction velocity* study, which assesses nerve damage or injury

endorphin: chemical substance in the brain that acts as an opiate; relieves pain by raising the body's pain threshold

enkephalin: similar to endorphin (see above)

eosinophilia myalgic syndrome (EMS): scleroderma-like thickening of fascia (see below) associated with high levels of circulating eosino-phils caused by a contaminant of l-tryptophan. Many patients with EMS develop fibromyalgia.

epidemiology: study of relationships between various factors that deter-mine who gets a disorder and how many people have it

epinephrine (adrenalin): a "nerve hormone" produced in the adrenal gland that acts as a neurotransmitter and stimulates the sympathetic nervous system

Epstein-Barr virus (EBV): a herpesvirus producing a mononucleosis-like illness that can lead to chronic fatigue syndrome

ergonomics: a discipline that studies the relationship between human factors, the design and operation of machines, behavior, and the physical environment

erythrocyte sedimentation rate (ESR): see **sedimentation rate**

excitatory amino acids: function as neurotransmitting chemicals in chronic pain. When they are blocked, fibromyalgia pain is relieved. Examples: glutamate and aspartate.

fascia: a layer of tissue between skin and muscle

female urethral syndrome (irritable bladder): persistent urge to void without evidence of infection, obstruction, stricture, or inflammation

fever: temperature above 99.6°F

fibromyalgia: chronic, widespread, amplified pain associated with fatigue, sleep disorder, tender points, and systemic symptoms

fibrositis: outdated term for fibromyalgia (see above); discarded since it implies inflammation, which is usually not present

flare: reappearance of symptoms; exacerbation

gamma-aminobutyric acid (GABA): an inhibitory neurotransmitter

gate theory: blocking or regulating transmission of pain impulses in the dorsal horn of the spinal column

gene: consisting of DNA, it is the basic unit of inherited information in our cells

Gulf War syndrome: fibromyalgia-like disorder among Gulf War (1991) veterans, probably caused by taking a combination of medicines meant to protect them from chemical warfare

handicap: job limitation; inability to do something

homeopathy: discipline based on the idea that symptoms can be eliminated by taking infinitesimal amounts of substances that, in large amounts, would produce the same symptoms

hormones: chemical made by the body, including thyroid-stimulating hormone, steroids, insulin, estrogen, progesterone, and testosterone

hyperalgesia: exaggerated response to a painful stimulus

hypermobility: laxity of ligaments allowing one to assume positions or undertake movements difficult for a normal person

hyperpathia: delayed or persistent pain from noxious stimuli

hypochondriasis: excessive preoccupation with the fear of having a serious disease based on misinterpretation of one or more bodily symptoms or signs

hypoglycemia: low blood sugar level

hypothalamic-pituitary-adrenal (HPA) axis: system by which a releasing hormone secreted by the hypothalamus induces the pituitary gland to secrete stimulating hormone, which in turn induces the adrenal glands to release steroid-related hormones

hypothalamus region of the brain that produces chemicals that result in the release of hormones

hypoxia: insufficient oxygen reaching a tissue, organ, or region of the body

hysteria: see **conversion reaction**

impairment: anatomic, physiologic, or psychological loss that leads to disability

incidence: rate at which a population develops a disorder

interferon: a protein with antiviral activity; has immune regulatory properties that can produce cognitive impairment and aching

interleukins: protein substances that are intercellular mediators of inflammation and the immune response

interstitial cystitis: a chronic inflammatory condition of the bladder

irritable bladder: see **female urethral syndrome**

irritable bowel syndrome: symptoms of abdominal distention, bloating, mucus-containing stools, and irregular bowel habits without an obvious cause

leaky gut syndrome: a controversial entity based on the belief that an overload of poisons overwhelms the liver's ability to detoxify, making the intestinal lining more permeable

ligament: connective-tissue "tether" attaching bones to other bones, giving them stability

limbic system: a collection of brain structures that influences endocrine and autonomic systems and affects motivational and mood states

livedo reticularis: lace-like pattern of small veins and capillaries visible on the skin

lupus (systemic lupus erythematosus [SLE]): autoimmune multisystemic disease caused by abnormal immune regulation resulting in tissue damage

Lyme disease: cause is a deer-borne tick that infects people with a bacterium; frequently associated with fibromyalgia and fatigue syndromes

lymphadenopathy: swollen, palpable lymph nodes

lymphocyte: type of white blood cell that fights infection and mediates the immune response

magnetic resonance imaging (MRI): modality by which a picture of a body region is obtained using powerful magnets; involves no radiation

melatonin: a substance made by the pineal gland of the brain that promotes sleep

migraine: a vascular headache

mitral valve prolapse: a floppy heart valve that can produce palpitations

multiple chemical sensitivity syndrome: controversial condition suggesting that chemicals in the environment produce symptoms and signs at levels not thought to be harmful

myalgia: pain in the muscles

myelinated fibers: fat-protein sheath surrounding nerve fibers

myoclonus: twitching of a muscle or a group of muscles

myofascial pain: discomfort in the muscles and fascia

myofascial pain syndrome: fibromyalgia-like pain limited to one region of the body; also known as regional myofascial pain

National Institutes of Health (NIH): federal government organization that funds medical research

neurally mediated hypotension: low blood pressure due to autonomic dysfunction

neurokinins: substances made by nerves having physiologic effects

neuropathic: pathology produced by compression, damage, or destruction of a nerve

neuropeptides: consist of short chemical sequences common to amino acids (a building block of protein) that have effects on one's perception of pain and can act as neurotransmitters

neuroplasticity: central brain sensitization that, if prolonged, produces phantom limb pain

neurotransmitters: chemical substances that transmit messages through nerves

nerve conduction velocity (NCV): measures the rate of nerve transmission and is usually part of an electromyogram (see above)

NMDA (*N*-methyl-D-aspartate) receptor: a neurotransmitter sensor or receptor different from that of opiates that interacts with excitatory amino acids (see above)

nociceptor: a nerve that receives and transmits painful stimuli. Nociception is the process through which stimuli from the periphery (skin, muscles, tissues) is transmitted to the central nervous system.

nonrestorative sleep: sleep after which one wakes up feeling unrefreshed

nonsteroidal anti-inflammatory drugs (NSAIDs): agents such as aspirin, ibuprofen, or naproxen that fight inflammation by blocking the actions of prostaglandin

norepinephrine: a "nerve hormone" produced in the adrenal gland that acts as a neurotransmitter and stimulates the autonomic nervous system

obsessive-compulsive disorder (OCD): persistent ideas or impulses; can include performing repetitive acts or perfectionistic tendencies

occupational therapy: uses ergonomics in designing tasks to fit the capabilities of the human body

opiates: specific group of narcotics

osteopath: a physician who is trained in performing specialized physical manipulative modalities

overuse syndrome: pain in muscles, ligaments, tendons, or joints from excessive activity in an area of the body

pain: an unpleasant sensation or emotional experience

palindromic rheumatism: intermittent swelling or inflammation of joints

palmar erythema: redness of the hands due to an autonomic reaction

parasympathetic nervous system: a division of the autonomic nervous system that blocks acetylcholine

paresthesia: sensation of numbness, tingling, burning, or prickling anywhere in the body

peripheral nervous system: nerves to and from the spinal cord that transmit sensation and motor reflexes

physiatrist: practitioner of physical medicine (see below)

physical medicine: medical specialty concerned with the principles of musculoskeletal, cardiovascular, and neurologic rehabilitation

physical therapist: allied health professional who assists patients with physical conditioning

pituitary: a gland in the brain that assists in the production of hormones

pleuritis: inflammation or irritation of the lining of the lung

polymyalgia rheumatica: an autoimmune disease of the joints and muscles seen in older patients with high sedimentation rates who have aching in their shoulders, upper arms, hips, and upper legs

polymyositis: an autoimmune inflammatory disorder of muscles

positron emission tomography (PET): an imaging technique that measures blood flow to, and often glucose uptake of, tissues

prednisone, prednisolone: synthetic steroids

premenstrual syndrome (PMS): the release of chemicals prior to menstruation, causing fluid retention, alterations in mood and behavior, and sometimes painful periods

prevalence: the number of people who have a condition or disorder per unit of population

primary fibromyalgia syndrome: fibromyalgia of unknown cause

prolactin: hormone that stimulates the secretion of breast milk

prostaglandins: physiologically active substances present in many tissues

protein: a collection of amino acids. Antibodies are proteins.

psychogenic rheumatism: complaints of joint pain for purposes of secondary gain

psychosomatic: when parts of the brain or mind influence functions of the body

rapid eye movement (REM) sleep: the part of sleep during which one may dream

Raynaud's disease: isolated Raynaud's phenomenon (see below); not part of any other disease

Raynaud's phenomenon: discoloration of the hands or feet (which turn blue, white, or red), especially with stress or cold temperatures; a feature of many autoimmune diseases

reactive hyperemia: increased blood flow to an area following prior interruption or compromise of circulation

referred pain: pain perceived as coming from an area different from its actual origin

reflex sympathetic dystrophy (RSD): type of fibromyalgia associated with sustained burning pain and swelling; also called complex regional pain syndrome, type 1

reflexology: form of alternative medicine based on the theory that specific areas of the ears, hands, and feet correspond to organs, glands, and nerves

regional myofascial syndrome: fibromyalgia pain limited to one region of the body; also known as myofascial pain syndrome

repetitive strain syndrome: when repetitive motions in a work environment produce strain or stress on an area of the body, as in carpal tunnel syndrome from excessive typing

restless legs syndrome: a form of periodic limb movement syndrome where legs suddenly shoot out, lift, jerk, or go into spasm. If this occurs during sleep, it is called sleep myoclonus.

seasonal affective disorder: light deprivation during winter months produces depression and fatigue

sedimentation rate: test that measures the rate of fall of red blood cells in a column of blood; high rates indicate inflammation or infection

selective serotonin reuptake inhibitors (SSRI): class of drugs that treat depression and pain by boosting serotonin levels

serotonin: a chemical that aids sleep, reduces pain, and influences mood and appetite. Derived from tryptophan and stored in blood platelets.

sicca syndrome: dry eyes. Can be due to decreased sympathetic nervous system activity, medication, or Sjögren syndrome (see below).

sick building syndrome: allergy and fibromyalgia-like symptoms complained of by more than one person with extreme sensitivity to environmental components in the same home or workplace

single photon emission computed tomography (SPECT): an imaging modality that measures uptake of one or more tracers by various tissues in the body

Sjögren syndrome: dry eyes, dry mouth, and arthritis observed in many autoimmune disorders or by itself (primary Sjögren syndrome)

sleep myoclonus: restless legs syndrome (see above) that occurs during sleep

slow wave sleep: phase of sleep not associated with dreaming but with alpha waves on an electroencephalogram (see above)

soft tissue rheumatism: musculoskeletal complaints relating to tendons, muscles, bursa, ligaments, and fascial tissues; includes fibromyalgia

somatization: conversion of anxiety and other psychological states into physical symptoms

somatomedin C: a form of growth hormone

somatotropin: growth hormone

spinoreticular tract: trail of nerves that conducts impulses to the brain and regulates the autonomic nervous system from the periphery

spinothalamic tract: trail of nerves that conveys impulses to the brain associated with touch, pain, and temperature

steroids: shortened term for corticosteroids, which are anti-inflammatory hormones produced either by the adrenal gland's cortex or synthetically

substance P: a neurotransmitter chemical that increases pain perception

sympathetic nervous system (SNS): a branch of the autonomic nervous system that regulates the release of norepinephrine (see above)

syndrome: a constellation of associated symptoms, signs, and laboratory findings

synovitis: inflammation of the tissues lining a joint

synovium: tissue lining a joint

taut band: a tight, rubber-band-like knot in the muscles

T cell: a lymphocyte responsible for immunologic memory

temporomandibular joint (TMJ) dysfunction syndrome: pain in the jaw joint associated with localized myofascial discomfort

tender point: area of tenderness in the muscles, tendons, bony prominences, or fat pads

tendon: structure that attaches muscle to bone

thalamus: an oval mass of gray matter in the brain that receives signals from nerve tracts in the spinal cord

Tietze syndrome: another term for costochondritis (see above)

tinnitus: ringing in the ears

titer: amount of a substance

tricyclics: a family of antidepressant drugs (e.g., amitriptyline [Elavil]) that relieve depression, promote restful sleep, relax muscles, and raise the pain threshold

trigger point: an area of muscle that, when touched, triggers a reaction of discomfort

tryptophan: an amino acid that can be broken down to serotonin

vaginismus: tightness of the vaginal muscles, which prevents or limits penetration during sexual intercourse

vertigo: malfunction of the vestibular (balance center) region of the ear, producing a sensation that everything around the sufferer is in motion

visceral hyperalgesia: pain amplification mediated by the parasympathetic nervous system, thought to cause irritable bowel and ulcer-like symptoms

vocational rehabilitation: training someone for an occupation that takes into account the person's educational background and physical skills, as well as his or her handicaps or impairments

vulvodynia: pain in the female genital area when infection, cancer, stricture, or inflammation has been ruled out

Index